A Sea of Broken Hearts

Patient Rights in a Dangerous, Profit-Driven Health Care System

by

John T. James, Ph.D

authorHOUSE®

AuthorHouse™
1663 Liberty Drive, Suite 200
Bloomington, IN 47403
www.authorhouse.com
Phone: 1-800-839-8640

First published by AuthorHouse 7/17/2007

ISBN: 978-1-4343-2136-7 (sc)

Library of Congress Control Number: 2007931697

Printed in the United States of America
Bloomington, Indiana

This book is printed on acid-free paper.

Cover Photo Courtesy Jim Cox

This book is dedicated in loving memory to Airman John Alexander James (September 24, 1982 – September 18, 2002). Alex, like hundreds of thousands of Americans each year, lost his life due to uninformed, inattentive, and unethical medical care. His story echoes the untold stories of other children, of brothers, fathers, and grandpas, of mothers, sisters, and grandmas, who died because of medical errors. Death came to them as an "adverse event."

Contents

Illustrations

Evidence

Glossary

American Board of Internal Medicine—an organization that certifies medical specialists, including most that practice various subspecialties of cardiology in the U.S.

angina—a transient pain caused when the heart muscles do not receive enough oxygen.

a**rrhythmia**—heartbeats observed on an ECG that occur too slowly or too quickly, not in a uniform pattern, or pass through the heart in abnormal pathways.

atrioventricular node—conducts electrical impulses from the atrium to the ventricles of the heart (Figure 1).

automated external defibrillator—a device capable of shocking the heart when it has begun to beat uselessly in small quavering beats called fibrillations.

cardiac catheterization—a method of examining the heart that involves insertion of a wire and small tubes into the heart; also called left heart catheterization in this book (Exhibit 10).

cardiac examination—a clinical procedure by which a physician can learn a great deal about a patient's heart without any sophisticated equipment.

cardiomyopathy—structural disease of the heart muscle.

clinical practice guidelines—widely disseminated procedures established by expert physician groups based on medical evidence. These procedures are to be used in caring for patients having conditions within the scope of the guideline.

current procedural terminology—a term used by the American Medical Association to identify discrete interventions or diagnostic practices that are developed to a specific level of usefulness in patient care.

depolarization—the portion of the heartbeat as seen on an ECG that signals the ventricles to contract abruptly (Figure 3).

diastole—the portion of the heartbeat when the heart refills with blood before the next contraction.

doctor (*v.*)—to falsify or change a record for the purpose of deception.

evidence-based medicine—the practice of patient care firmly guided by scientific knowledge based on the best-available medical data and conclusions.

electroencephalogram—a non-invasive technique in which sensors placed on the head are used to analyze the brain's electrical activity in response to stimuli.

hypokalemia—a medical condition in which the patient has a serum potassium level below 3.6 millimoles per liter (mmol/L).

hypokalemic cardiomyopathy—cellular injury and scarring of the heart muscle caused by potassium depletion.

hypomagnesemia—a medical condition in which the patient has a serum magnesium level below 1.8 mmol/L.

iatrogenic—caused by a physician.

informed consent—the process by which a physician communicates to a patient the reasons and alternatives for an invasive medical procedure, after which the patient acknowledges that he understands his choices.

invasive medical procedure—a medical procedure involving surgical tools from which the patient could receive serious injury or be killed.

ischemia—reduced blood flow and oxygen availability to tissues.

loop monitor—a device about the size of a cigarette lighter that is inserted under the skin of the chest. It records heartbeats of the wearer when the wearer activates it.

maintenance of certification—a term used by medical boards to identify the process by which specialists they certify retain their certification. It typically involves a demonstration of continued practice in the specialty, a self assessment, and completion of a secure examination.

maintenance of competency—a term I will use interchangeably with maintenance of certification. Physicians much prefer that "certification" rather than "competency" be used.

master diagnostic technician—an automobile mechanic who has demonstrated competency in identifying the causes of mechanical problems with a vehicle and repairing the problem.

medical literature—periodic journals containing peer-reviewed scientific and clinical studies that aid our understanding of the causes and treatment of disease.**myocarditis**—an inflammation of the heart muscle.

National Council on Potassium in Clinical Practice—an expert group assembled to define clinical practice guidelines for replacement of potassium in patients who are depleted in this electrolyte.

pacemaker—a device that generates electrical signals through wires implanted in the heart to override the signals coming from the sinoatrial node of the heart.

peer review—a process by which scientific and medical manuscripts are reviewed by at least 2 experts selected by a journal editor in the field of the research. These experts criticize the manuscript and recommend to the journal editor whether or not to publish the paper. The criticisms are passed along to the author of the manuscript; the names of the reviewers are not.

physician in training—in Texas this is a person who has received a medical education from a "suitable" medical school and has passed the first 2 stages of a 3-part examination series. Such physicians are under the supervision of a fully-licensed physician and at the end of training are expected to take the 3rd part of the examination.

repolarization—the portion of the cardiac cycle, as seen on an ECG, in which the heart prepares for the next heartbeat. It extends from the S to the end of the T wave (Figure 3).

serum—the yellowish fluid remaining after the clot and cells are separated from blood.

sinoatrial node—the bundle of nerve cells where electrical impulses originate and enter the atrium of the heart (Figure 1).

statin—a therapeutic drug that reduces synthesis of cholesterol and increases removal of low-density lipoprotein from the bloodstream to reduce the risk of coronary artery disease.

syncope—loss of consciousness for a brief period of time.

systole—the part of the cardiac cycle when the heart squeezes blood into the arteries of the body and lungs.

valve (in heart)—one of the round openings with 2 or 3 flaps that control the flow of blood into and out of the heart.

ventricular fibrillation—quivering of the heart muscle in a way that moves very little blood and puts the patient's life in immediate danger (Figure 5).

ventricular tachycardia—inappropriately rapid beating of the ventricles of the heart. In medical shows on TV, the actors refer to this as V-tach. It can degenerate into ventricular fibrillation (Figure 5).

Abbreviations

ABIM	American Board of Internal Medicine
ABMS	American Board of Medical Specialties
ACE	angiotensin converting enzyme
AED	automated external defibrillator
AMA	American Medical Association
AIDS	acquired immune deficiency syndrome
BPM	beats per minute (of the heart)
CEO	chief executive officer
CME	continuing medical education
CPG	clinical practice guideline
CPR	cardiopulmonary resuscitation
DHHS	Department of Health and Human Services
DPRC	Disciplinary Process Review Committee (the group within the TMB that is responsible for disciplining physicians and other licensed medical personnel)
ECG (or EKG)	electrocardiogram
EEG	electroencephalogram
EMT	emergency medical technician
EP	electrophysiology
ER	emergency room
FAA	Federal Aviation Administration
FOIA	Freedom of Information Act
HF	Heart failure
HIV	human immunodeficiency virus
ICD	implantable cardioverter-defibrillator
IOM	Institute of Medicine (of the National Academy of Sciences)
IV	intravenous
JAMA	*Journal of the American Medical Association*
JCAHO	Joint Commission on Accreditation of Healthcare Organizations
LQTS	long QT syndrome
MMOL/L	millimoles per liter (a measure of the concentration of an electrolyte)

MOC	Maintenance of Certification
MRI	magnetic resonance image (imaging)
MS	milliseconds
PIT	Physician in Training
PVC	pre-ventricular contraction (or complex)
QT	ECG interval from the start of the Q wave to the end of the T wave
QTc	QT interval corrected for heart rate
QTd	the maximum dispersion (difference) in QT values from different tracings on an ECG
SCD	sudden cardiac death
TMB	Texas Medical Board (formerly the TSBME)
TSBME	Texas State Board of Medical Examiners

Cardiology Tool Box: Dog-ear this page so you can find your tools. The application of each tool is given in Chapter 1.

1. The **electrical system** that stimulates the ventricles to contract passes through the ventricular septum of the heart, a wall of tissue between the left and right ventricles.

2. The **nervous system** and hormones control the rate at which the heart beats.

3. **Potassium**, an electrolyte which is highly concentrated inside living cells, is critical for normal heart function.

4. **Arrhythmias** that can be seen on an electrocardiogram (ECG) include a prolonged QT interval and pre-ventricular contractions (PVCs). Potassium depletion can cause the QT interval to increase and can increase the frequency of PVCs.

5. **Potassium depletion** can be caused by a person doing demanding exercise in a hot climate, especially if the person has a low dietary intake of potassium-rich foods.

6. **Magnesium deficiency** and potassium deficiency often go hand in hand because their sources in the diet are similar.

7. **Low potassium and low magnesium** in serum are independently associated with an increase in the prevalence of PVCs.

8. **The gateway to sudden cardiac death** is through PVCs, especially if the patient has structural injuries; however, most PVCs are harmless.

9. **Death of cells** causes release of enzymes and potassium into the blood.

10. **Ventricular fibrillation**, a life-threatening arrhythmia, can occur when ventricles fail to receive and respond to normal electrical impulses. A prolonged QT interval increases the risk of ventricular fibrillation.

11. **A heart-rate corrected QT interval** (QTc) on an ECG is abnormal if it is above 450 milliseconds (ms).

12. **Written communication** is the medical standard for helping patients manage their health risks. Physicians must identify **risk factors** in medical data and in the patient's lifestyle, and then help the patient manage these risk factors.

13. **Informed consent** has been defined by the American Medical Association (AMA) to include a thorough discussion of the purpose of an invasive procedure, the alternatives to doing the procedure, and the risks of injury or death from the procedure.

14. A high **QT dispersion** (wide difference) in the QT values in the tracings on an ECG is a risk factor for sudden cardiac death.

Note to the Reader

The practice of medicine is not a precise undertaking, so there is always room for contrary opinions that may be more or less based on evidence. I am asking you to believe me over several cardiologists who treated or reviewed the treatment of my son. I have accepted information contained in peer-reviewed medical literature and major cardiology textbooks as true. By doing that, I am trusting that the system that controls the quality of information published in medical journals and textbooks is robust. Often I give the name of the medical journal I have used as a source so that you will have increased confidence in the information I cite. Occasionally, I have referenced newspaper articles to make non-technical points addressed by a columnist.

If you were to ask a cardiologist if I have made mistakes herein, he would find some; however, just ask him to back up his "expert" opinion with publications in the peer-reviewed medical literature. And then ask him what continuing medical education in cardiology he did last year and when he was last evaluated for competency; ask him if he uses the AMA definition of informed consent for his patients, how he practices evidence-based medicine, and when he last doctored a patient's medical record.

Key points I want to emphasize in the text have been highlighted in bold italics. For the most part I have tried to keep my grief and anger out of this book. Inevitably, both show through at times and, against the advice of some, I have decided to leave these in place. Death of a child when that child should never have died fosters grief and anger, and I would be "faking it" to purge these emotions from my story.

Acknowledgments

I wish to thank many colleagues and neighbors who took time to review this book in various stages of its development and to Dr. Jane Krauhs for her excellent and patient editing of the later manuscripts.

Preface

I am fearful of writing the story you are about to read. As I begin putting words into my computer, I wonder if I'll be able to finish telling it to you. At a minimum I will be revisited often by the grief monster that has stalked me since the day in September 2002 when my 19-year-old son Alex died. At times I can keep that monster at a safe distance, but all too often I am suddenly caught in its net and pulled into profound anguish. I have learned to let the monster feast on my heart until I am numb and my spiritual blood has run out, and then I can push it away for a little while longer. Telling Alex's story, and knowing that *millions* of other Americans have suffered and died over the years because of their medical care, invites the monster's return.

No one in the world wishes more than I do that it could be said that my son received reasonable care at the hands of his cardiologists. Alex was in their "care" for 5 days and endured all the testing they asked for, yet they gave him no diagnosis or treatment. Only 2½ weeks after seeing his last physician, he was lying on the running trail at his university with the last breath of life gone from his body. You and those you love are likely to have their lives in the hands of a cardiologist someday. Will you fear that cardiologist, or will you trust him? I trusted my son's cardiologists, and that's the biggest mistake I have ever made. As the mystery of his death unfolded I found an incredible conspiracy of ignorance and complicity among other cardiologists and physicians.

You might imagine that the chances that you will be personally affected by a medical error are small, but they are not small. In the year after Alex died 685,000 Americans died of heart disease and another 557,000 died of cancer. A convincing case can be made that the next leading cause of death in America is the medical care system (I am not the first to make this assertion). These are errors of omission and commission, and not all are preventable. Estimates in leading medical journals and reviews are as follows: deaths of outpatients due to therapeutic drug use, 199,000; deaths of hospitalized patients due to therapeutic drug use, 106,000; deaths of heart failure patients that could have been avoided by administering beta-blockers, 100,000; deaths due to hospital-acquired infections, 80,000; and deaths due to medical errors documented in medical records of inpatients, 98,000. No doubt there is some overlap in the deaths covered by these estimates, but it is clear that medical errors easily constitute the 3rd leading cause of death in the U.S., well ahead of the 158,000 who die from cerebral vascular disease. I'll write more about the basis of these estimates later. *If you know someone who died of heart disease or cancer, then you know someone who died from a medical error. The only difference is that the American medical system is adept at concealing its mistakes, so you are not aware that that person died of a medical error.* The American medical community knows that these errors exist, but patients do not.

I am not a cardiologist, but I am a Ph.D. pathologist and a board-certified toxicologist. During my son's illness I knew very little cardiology and had no choice except to trust his doctors. I never set out to discover that they had given him awful medical care. Their last recommendation was that he should be tested for a genetic disease, and when he died a few weeks later it became very important that I obtain his medical records and determine if his younger sister and brother were at risk. When I received those records, I immediately saw that they contained false statements and were grossly incomplete. That started my journey from one troubling discovery to another as I compared Alex's records, which I eventually obtained in complete form, with information in medical texts and medical literature. I have had the benefit of access to a medical library and to discussions with physicians working for the same federal agency as I do. Typically, they were uncomfortable discussing the possible mistakes of other physicians.

As I researched my son's illness, I came to realize that the standard for medical care in Texas, and much of the U.S., is far below what patients would accept if they knew the situation. Physicians define standards for treatment in major medical journals and in consensus recommendations from their professional societies, yet they fail to hold each other to these standards of patient care. *Clueless patients continue to allow physicians to set and enforce their own standards of care.* As a patient, or prospective patient, you must seize control of the standards of patient care by supporting effective legislation, NOW. This legislation must demand that all physicians in life-critical specialties demonstrate and maintain knowledge in their specialty for as long as they practice. Furthermore, all physicians must openly share medical records with their patients and never perform an invasive procedure without genuine informed consent. The secrecy that shrouds the process of dealing with complaints against physicians must disappear. Physicians must never be allowed to get away with falsifying medical records. The medical boards in Texas and other states must be reconstituted so that physicians cannot dominate the deliberations. *In short: the medical care in this country must become transparent and patient-focused rather than physician-focused. One of the best ways to achieve this is a patients' bill of rights.*

Physicians (and other dedicated medical personnel) are a precious resource to be cherished and respected. They originated from the best and brightest among us and most started their careers with the purpose of learning to heal the afflictions of others. Most have been highly successful in achieving that goal. More than a few have not.

I offer this book with my deepest apologies to those physicians who have worked tirelessly for a safe, patient-centered medical system, maintained state-of-the-art knowledge in their medical specialty, practiced evidence-based medicine, taken the time to thoroughly evaluate medical test data on their patients, offered genuine informed consent to their patients, never "doctored" their records, and consistently reported their colleagues who may have become a danger to their patients' safety.

Prologue
September 15, 2002: The Longest Drive

I am driving from Clear Lake City on the southeast side of Houston to central Texas, in the middle of the night. I am trying to adhere to the "Texas Ten" as I push my old Camry through the streetlight glare, noting that even at this hour I-45 and I-10 are still carrying many aggressive drivers. My thoughts are hardly on the freeway. An hour ago I received the worst phone call of my life. My wife had taken the call and said that Dr. Wilson was on the line and his call was for me. I have a physician friend from church named Dr. Wilson, so I assumed it was he on the line. Once I reached the phone I quickly realized that this was not that Dr. Wilson, it was the cardiologist, Dr. Wilson, from the city where my son was starting his junior year as a college student. He told me that Alex was found collapsed on the campus and that it had taken 3 shocks from the paramedics' paddles to get his heart restarted. He was on a respirator in a deep and unresponsive coma. Dr. Wilson said that his prognosis was not good.

When I got off the phone I carefully relayed the grave news to my wife, not conveying to her the terrible prognosis that her firstborn son had received. How could I tell the woman I love more than anything that her precious son was probably dying? Alex had been born almost 20 years ago after my wife had had 3 miscarriages. After he was conceived, she spent several months in bed to preserve his life. I can remember all too well the day the ultrasound revealed a tiny baby with a vigorously beating heart inside my wife's womb. I can remember the excitement we shared when Alex wiggled in her tummy, pushing waves across her abdomen. And so on this night I told her that her son had collapsed again and that he had not recovered consciousness as he had done a few weeks earlier. I was driving there to see what I could do.

As I passed out of the glare of Houston and headed northwest on highway 290, the sky finally darkened and I began to think about my athletic son who was clinging to life in a hospital so far away. It was now past midnight, September 16, 2002. I decided that I could push the old Camry to a speed just below 80 mph; there were few drivers on the dark road. Alex was young and maybe his vigorous lifestyle would enable him to recover consciousness and be well again. What had gone wrong?

My thoughts turned to the day he was born in Columbia, Maryland. He was a most precious child because of the difficulty my wife had with this pregnancy. He was born about 8 AM on September 24, 1982. He had a robust weight, but before long he developed jaundice. In those days the mother and child were not separated to control medical costs, so my wife was in the hospital for 6 days waiting for the lights in the incubator to destroy the bilirubin that was turning him yellow. At the time I was in graduate school in pathology and I knew that my son's bilirubin levels were approaching levels where he would need an exchange transfusion to protect his brain. Bilirubin can damage the brain if it crosses the blood-brain barrier. We had even started discussing his possible transfer to St. Agnes Hospital, where such transfusions were done. Fortunately his bilirubin peaked just under the level where he would have to go for a transfusion, and he recovered.

Life with Alex as a toddler was a treat. He was curious, smart, and easily disposed to giggling at any sort of antics. He especially loved to play in water. The beach was heaven for him. Before too long he was joined in our family by his baby sister Laura. She was, like most siblings, a target for conflict and for love. She was just 20 months younger than Alex and they had grown up together in Maryland and later in Texas. The day he went off to college she presented him with a framed collage showing pictures of their growing up together. Her message to him was, "I love you brother, don't forget all the good times we shared as you go off to college." I had made the turn off Route 290 and had gone a little way on Texas Route 6. I was passing Texas A&M University, where Laura had just started college. I would pass within a few miles of the tiny dorm room where she was sleeping. Only a few weeks before, I had emailed her Alex's good news that his doctors had given him a clean bill of health. I knew her heart would be shattered over the news that her brother could die.

I continued to push the Camry northwest past Bryan, being careful to slow down in the small towns that clung to existence along the route between there and my destination. My mind turned back to the innocent days in Maryland when Alex and Laura were little children. We enjoyed fishing in the pond behind our house, swinging in the park, playing in the snow when it came, and worshiping at a small church called Wesley Grove United Methodist Church. In the first Christmas season in Alex's life, he played baby Jesus and his mama was Mary in the church's production of the Christmas story. In years to come, their mama taught and directed the preschool, referring to her 2 children as the "aggie twins." This was because they could aggravate their mama with their antics and conflicts.

Laura had just turned 5 and Alex was almost 7 when we moved to Texas in our Mazda 323. We also moved Alex's hamster named Spike and Buffy, the small white dog I had bought for my wife after her last miscarriage. Laura had managed to step on some glass just before we left

Maryland and the gash, which required 6 stitches, gave her a lot of pain, which she readily shared with the rest of her family. We were coming to Texas so that I could work for NASA at Johnson Space Center in Clear Lake City, Texas. We quickly found a church in the area that was 10 times the size of the one we left, but it was full of warm people. I thought about praying for my son again on this dark night. I had prayed as I held the hands of the dozen folks in my bible study 2 weeks before, "God, please guard Alex's health and preserve his soul." The next day I had gotten the good news from him about his clean bill of health. At the time I thought my prayer had been answered! What had happened, God? Why was I now driving to a distant hospital to see my dying son? I was angry at God, very angry, but I said a quiet prayer anyway.

Alex's years in Clear Lake were full of baseball, swimming, band, science fairs, church choir, and church mission trips. Except for a bout with mononucleosis when he was about 10 years old, his health had been excellent. About this time in his life, he and his family were surprised by the birth of his little brother Austen. This little boy had indeed been a surprise to Alex's mama and me. At first Alex was afraid to hold Austen for fear of dropping him, but before long he was holding Austen and as the years passed they became great friends despite their 9-year difference in age. I thought one of Alex's strengths was that he could be a fierce competitor with his friends, yet he could play football or basketball with Austen and his friends with restraint so that no one got hurt. How would this little boy who loved his big brother beyond measure deal with his brother's serious, probably fatal illness? The inky darkness of central Texas began to give way to light along the horizon as I approached the city.

My route to the hospital took me through the campus of the college. I looked over at the dark music building where Alex's mama and I had said goodbye to him only 2 years before. This had been a long, painful day as we did a few superficial activities with the marching band community and then suddenly it was time to hug Alex with all our love, turn our backs on him, and walk to our car. Friends warned us not to look back, and my wife and I held hands, and we did not look back. Our son was in the care of his university and of the city community.

Alex's start in college had been a mixed experience for him. He had done well in his classes, but the new bicycle he bought before going to college was stolen within a few weeks and then his old Blazer was broken into in one of the parking lots. Glass from the passenger window was scattered throughout the front seat and floor. His messages and telephone calls to us (his parents) did not reveal the deep loneliness and faith struggles he expressed in an email to his aunt at the start of his second semester.

"I haven't told anyone this yet, but I have had a really tough time meeting people and making friends. I have prayed about it, but from what I can tell, nothing has happened to change the current situation, which is the fact that I have no friends here at all. It is hard to get out of bed every day knowing that I will go to class and study 6 or seven hours the rest of the day, and not have anyone ask me how things are going, or if I want to go to a movie, or anything...I have also been struggling in my faith. The religion class that I am currently enrolled in is not helping me at all; in fact, it made things worse, but in order to graduate, I have to take the class!...I definitely believe Jesus is Christ and he died to save our sins, but I do not know what to believe as far as the details of his life are concerned..."

I could also see parts of the "Jogging Trail," where I knew my son enjoyed running. Somewhere on this trail he had collapsed just a few hours before. I pointed the Camry through the silence that shrouded the city at this time of morning, and found the hospital, and then I found my son's room. This book is not about grief, so I will not attempt to share with you the story of the 3 days while my son was dying. There are no words to capture what one feels as he watches his 19-year-old son die and watches those he loves go through the deepest of anguish. In those 3 days my entire extended family gathered in Hospital 1 to support those of us closest to my son. God came to us through our church friends and our ministers, and the people of the college community poured out their kindness on us. In the late evening of September 18, 2002, I was the one who had to announce to the group that Alex had died.

His death sent me on a journey that I never sought. I would discover that his death was totally unnecessary, and that there was no means to hold his pitiful physicians accountable for their errors. I share that journey with you, along with some general information about doctors, so that you will personally take action before you die in the hands of an incompetent cardiologist or other doctor. The time to act is not when you need a physician, it is long before that, when incompetent physicians can be identified and disciplined effectively to protect innocent people from dying because of their doctor's incompetence. If incompetent physicians continue to practice, then you are likely to encounter the same "standard of medical care" received by my dead son.

Chapter 1
Your Cardiology Tool Box

You will need a few basic cardiology tools to help you solve the mystery of Alex's death after his heart had received so much evaluation by cardiologists. The knowledge you need can be gleaned from sources intended primarily for non-physicians, although at times you will need a tool formed from the medical literature intended for cardiologists. Some of these tools will be "sharpened" later.

How Your Heart Works

Your heart is a beautifully-timed, 4-chamber, muscular pump that contracts more than 2 *billion* times in an ordinary lifetime (Figure 1). The smaller right side of the heart receives unoxygenated blood from the body and propels it to the lungs to receive oxygen from the air and have carbon dioxide removed. The more powerful left side of the heart receives oxygenated blood from the lungs and propels it into the body through arteries branching to capillaries, which supply oxygen to the tissues and receive carbon dioxide as a waste product of metabolism in the tissues. Veins return the oxygen-depleted blood to the right side of the heart, and the process is repeated again. A series of 4 valves inside the heart controls the direction of blood flow. If you rode on a red blood cell as the heart moves it along, you would visit the following places in this order: right atrium, right ventricle, lungs, left atrium, left ventricle, arteries of the body, capillaries of the body, veins of the body, right atrium, and so on. Heart muscles require large amounts of oxygen as they do their work; the coronary arteries, branching from the aorta (leading out of the left ventricle), deliver this oxygenated blood to the cardiac muscles.

Heartbeats consist of 2 general features: the sequence of muscular contractions that send blood through the heart chambers and the frequency of those contractions. The sequence of contractions has 3 phases: diastole (filling of the chambers with blood as they expand), atrial systole (squeezing of blood from the atria into their respective ventricles), and ventricular systole (squeezing of the blood to the lungs or general circulation). The timing of atrial systole is determined by electrical waves of excitation, or impulses, that originate in the sinoatrial node located in the right atrium. Ventricular systole is initiated by an impulse from the atrioventricular node, which receives an impulse from the sinoatrial node (see Figure 1). The electrical pathway from the sinoatrial node passes through the Bundle of His, and cells called Purkinje fibers rapidly distribute impulses to the muscular portion of the heart. The Bundle of His is divided into left and right branches, which spread down the left and right sides, respectively, of the wall dividing the right and left ventricles (septum). The muscle cells of the ventricles contract immediately after the impulse reaches them; this is called *depolarization.* Between contractions the heart muscle *repolarizes,* and then each cell relaxes in preparation for its next contraction.

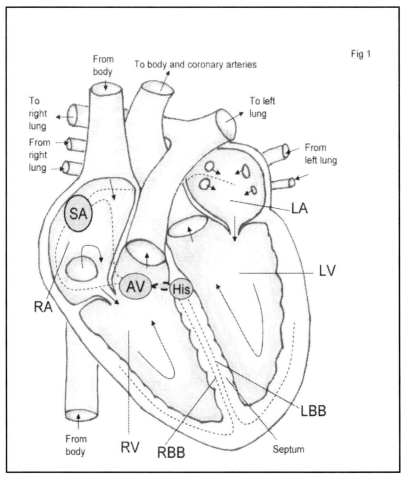

Figure 1. Flow of blood in the heart is indicated by arrows and its basic electrical system is shown with dotted lines. The blood-pumping chambers are the right atrium (RA), right ventricle (RV), left atrium (LA), and left ventricle (LV). In the electrical system the sinoatrial (SA) node sends impulses to the atrioventricular node (AV), which sends impulses to the Bundle of His. Then the signal for the ventricles to contract passes through the left bundle branch (LBB) and right bundle branch (RBB) in the septum.

Tool 1: The electrical system that stimulates the ventricles of the heart to contract normally passes through the ventricular septum, the wall of tissue between the left and right ventricles. Put this tool in a safe place where you can find it later. It may help you identify a killer.

The frequency of heartbeats would be about 100 beats per minute (bpm) without external control of the rate by the nervous system. The parasympathetic nervous system slows the beat so that at rest the frequency is only 60-70 bpm, and during times of greater need for blood, the sympathetic nervous system can speed up the frequency of beats to more than 200 bpm (at least in young people). During exercise or times of extreme stress, release of the hormones epinephrine and norepinephrine from the adrenal glands (on top of the kidneys) also helps increase the frequency of heartbeats and divert blood to the muscles and away from less critical parts such as the digestive system and skin. The heart of a well-conditioned athlete at rest can beat at frequencies below 40 bpm.

Tool 2: The nervous system and hormones control the rate of beating of the heart.

Another important facet of normal heart function is the proper balance of the blood chemicals called "electrolytes" that the heart muscles need for contracting as electrical signals are sent to them. The amount of the electrolyte potassium outside a heart muscle cell affects the stability of the muscle cell membrane, which is the soap-bubble-like surface separating the inside of each cell from its surroundings. As the extracellular potassium decreases, the ability of this membrane to allow potassium to go through it decreases and the magnitude of depolarization increases; low extracellular potassium is called *hypokalemia* and is clinically evident by a low potassium concentration in the plasma or serum.

Tool 3: Potassium, which is highly concentrated inside all living cells of the body, is crucial to normal heart function (Figure 2).

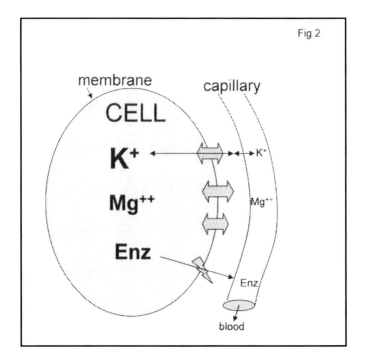

Figure 2: Cell showing enzymes (Enz), electrolytes (K⁺ and Mg⁺⁺) and membrane receptors (double arrows). Potassium (K⁺), magnesium (Mg⁺⁺), and enzymes are highly concentrated inside cells. With each "beat" of a heart muscle cell, potassium passes in and out of the cell through receptors located on the cell's membrane. There are various types of potassium receptors. When the membrane ruptures, specific enzymes escape from the cell and are elevated in the serum; detection of elevated enzymes in the serum can identify the organ in which cell death is occurring.

In some cases hypokalemia can increase the interval from the start of depolarization to the end of repolarization, prolonging the QT interval (Olgin and Zipes, 2001). The QT interval is shown in an electrocardiogram (ECG) (Figure 3). Hypokalemia is also associated with an increase in the frequency of premature ventricular complexes (PVCs) (Tsuji et al., 1994). PVCs are contractions of the ventricles that are not initiated through the normal electrical pathways shown in Figure 1; instead these originate in the ventricles themselves and are called "ventricular ectopic beats" by cardiologists. Sometimes a person can sense the pounding beat that follows a PVC, but most often one cannot. To quote a cardiology text (Richardson et al., 1998): *"It is clear why physicians monitor plasma potassium so carefully!"* Other electrolytes such as sodium, magnesium, and calcium are also important to cardiac function, but potassium is critical for normal heart function.

Tool 4: Potassium depletion can cause a dangerous increase in the QT interval and increase the prevalence of PVCs (Figure 3).

This tool enables you to make a simple connection between abnormal features in an ECG (called arrhythmias) and measurements of electrolytes such as potassium. Later you can sharpen this tool using a widely-published medical guideline that an informed cardiologist would have applied to Alex's care.

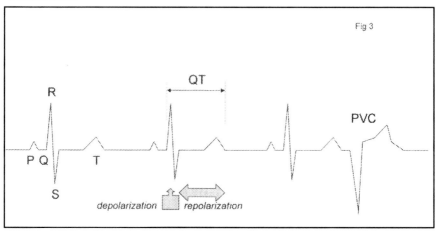

Figure 3. Typical ECG showing QT interval, re/depolarization and a PVC.

Electrolytes, especially magnesium and potassium, are essential for normal heart function. We can gain insight into the importance of potassium to normal heart function and causes of hypokalemia from a review article in the *New England Journal of Medicine* written by a physician (Gennari, 1998) simply titled "Hypokalemia." Quoting from that article, "Drugs prescribed by physicians are the most common causes of hypokalemia...In the absence of an inciting drug, hypokalemia can result from inadequate intake, or from abnormal losses." The article provides a table listing the drugs that cause hypokalemia, including epinephrine, bronchodilators, diuretics, high dose antibiotics, and one of my favorites, caffeine. Citing a research study the article states, "The caffeine in a few cups of coffee can decrease serum potassium by as much as 0.4 millimole per liter (mmol/L)." Gennari asserts in one place that hypokalemia from inadequate dietary intake is rarely the cause of hypokalemia; however, later when discussing potassium replacement he states, "The safest approach to minimizing [the risk of] hypokalemia is to ensure adequate dietary potassium intake."

Excessive losses of potassium may occur because of kidney dysfunction or discharge of potassium in the stool, especially if diarrhea is present.

One kind of loss not mentioned in the review article is that from copious sweating caused by intense, sustained exercise in a hot climate. Years ago significant losses of potassium were demonstrated in military recruits participating in basic training under hot conditions. Knochel et al. (1972) showed in research published in the *Journal of Clinical Investigation* that "Although sweating was the avenue by which the [potassium] deficit occurred, daily excretion of potassium into the urine when each subject was maximally deficient…was inappropriately high for potassium-depleted subjects…We observed that potassium depletion occurred only in men training in hot climates." Despite the potassium depletion, "No subject became frankly hypokalemic." The range of average plasma potassium in the test subjects varied from 3.5 to 4.1 mmol/L during training.

Tool 5: Loss of electrolytes, especially potassium, is likely when a patient has been doing demanding exercise for weeks to months in a hot climate. Adequate dietary intake of potassium can reduce the risk of potassium depletion.

Gennari (1998) points out that magnesium depletion often coexists with potassium depletion and that replenishment of magnesium improves the coexistent potassium deficit. Ordinary foods that are good sources of magnesium are similar to those that are good sources of potassium. For example, nuts, beans, and whole grains have the highest contents of both electrolytes. Fruits, vegetables, and meats (except chicken) are also good sources of both. Most of these are foods that are recommended in a healthy diet.

Tool 6: Potassium and magnesium deficiency often go hand-in-hand because their sources in the diet are similar.

The finding that low serum potassium or, independently, low serum magnesium is correlated with an increased prevalence of PVCs underscores the importance of these electrolytes to heart function (Tsuji et al., 1994). The rationale for Tsuji's study, which was published in the *American Journal of Cardiology*, was as follows: "Since arrhythmias caused by serum electrolyte depletion can be prevented by electrolyte repletion, it is important to investigate the relations between electrolyte levels and arrhythmia risk." Using a carefully screened normal population of more than 3,000 adults, the investigators found that the prevalence of PVCs was 77% higher in persons whose serum potassium level was below 4.4 mmol/L than in those with a level above 4.9 mmol/L, and the group whose serum magnesium level was below 1.8 mmol/L had a 71% higher prevalence of PVCs than the group with a magnesium level above 2.0 mmol/L.

Tool 7: Low potassium and low magnesium in the blood are each independently associated with an increase in the prevalence of PVCs.

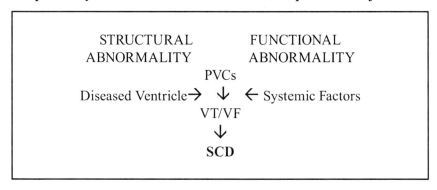

Figure 4. PVCs as the gateway through which structural and functional abnormalities lead to sudden cardiac death (SCD) (Myerburg et al, 1989). Diagram is simplified and focused on my son's heart "abnormalities." Further resolution is provided in Figure 6. Figure 5 shows what VT (ventricular tachycardia) and VF (ventricular fibrillation) look like on an ECG.

Although most PVCs are harmless, they are generally understood to be the gateway to sudden cardiac death (SCD) (Myerburg et al., 1989) (Figure 4). In an article published in the *American Journal of Cardiology* entitled "A biological approach to sudden cardiac death; structure, function and cause," Myerburg and his coauthors show how functional deficits such as electrolyte imbalances can interact with structural deficits such as ventricular disease to cause PVCs, which lead to subsequent ventricular fibrillation (rapid quivering of the ventricle), followed by sudden death. This is distinct from the more common "heart attack" caused by blockage of coronary arteries. Myerburg's work in this area was sufficiently important to be included as a chapter in a major cardiology textbook edited by 3 other cardiologists and entitled *"Heart Disease, A Textbook of Cardiovascular Medicine"* (Myerburg and Castellanos, 1997). The chapter appeared again in the 2001 edition of the same textbook (Myerburg and Castellanos, 2001). Just in case your cardiologist has not been reading cardiology textbooks and does not know the basics about the importance of electrolytes, now you do.

Tool 8: You should now be aware of the connection between electrolyte imbalances such as low potassium and/or magnesium and the appearance of PVCs in a patient's ECG. PVCs in turn can be the gateway to sudden cardiac death, especially if the patient has structural deficits. Later you can use this "master tool" to understand what Alex's cardiologists were unable to deduce from his medical tests.

Structural Diseases of the Heart and Their Symptoms

The heart is a complex organ on which high demands are made throughout life. As you might imagine, many types of diseases can affect the ability of the heart to perform its job of circulating blood to the lungs and body tissues. These diseases can be clinically silent (no overt symptoms) until the moment of death or they can have a slow onset with gradual erosion of cardiac performance spread over years or even decades. The diseases may be caused by genetic disorders or lifestyle choices that increase the risk of heart disease. Often, genetic and lifestyle choices combine to precipitate and/or accelerate heart disease. In addition, external factors such as electrolyte imbalances can destroy the ability of the heart to perform its normal job of pumping blood and can cause structural injury to the heart. An attractive picture book edited by Charles B. Clayman, M.D. (The American Medical Association [AMA], 1989) and published by the Reader's Digest Association, Pleasantville, New York provides an understandable overview of heart diseases for non-physicians. Below I will summarize selected information from that book, supplementing some areas with information extracted from two issues of the *Mayo Clinic Health Letter*, which is published monthly by the Mayo Foundation for Medical Education and Research, Rochester, Minnesota. *As I read these two sources for non-physicians I have to ask myself if some cardiologists I know of, particularly those associated with my son's treatment, would substantially improve their knowledge of cardiology if only they knew this information intended for laypersons.*

Coronary Artery Disease

The heart muscle requires a high blood flow to deliver oxygen and nutrients to it efficiently so that it can do its job of pumping blood to the lungs and body. That blood flow is delivered to the heart muscle by the coronary arteries. As we age, most of us develop a narrowing of the coronary arteries called atherosclerosis. As the narrowing progresses over the years, one may occasionally feel pain spreading into the neck, through the back, or down the left arm during exertion as the coronary arteries fail to deliver enough blood; this is called angina. If the angina worsens, that is increases in intensity or frequency, or occurs with less exertion, the risk that a heart attack will occur within a few months increases. A heart attack occurs when the lumen (hollow interior) of a coronary artery becomes obstructed and it can no longer deliver oxygenated, nutrient-rich blood to the heart muscle, resulting in death of some of the muscle. This obstruction of the artery lumen is thought to occur when a plaque along the artery wall splits and precipitates clot formation in the lumen. This is why anticoagulants such as aspirin and clot busters such as thrombolysins are essential treatments within the first few hours after a heart attack.

Each year, about one million Americans have a heart attack. As heart tissue dies from lack of oxygen, cardiac enzymes, which are concentrated inside the heart cells, are released into the blood. Other cellular contents such as potassium and magnesium are also released into the blood (Figure 2, page 4). If the heart is so seriously damaged that it cannot deliver oxygenated blood to bodily tissues, then enzymes, potassium, and magnesium are released from this tissue as it dies from lack of oxygen.

Tool 9: Death of cells in the body causes release of enzymes and some electrolytes into the blood. This tool will be valuable as you consider one of the superficial evaluations provided by a cardiologist who examined my son's medical records.

Arrhythmias

Heart rhythm disturbances (arrhythmias) are generally a manifestation of one of the structural deficits noted above, genetic disease, an electrolyte imbalance, hormonal disturbances, or some combination of these. Cardiologists describe arrhythmias in terms of the features they can observe on an ECG and their ability to surmise the anatomical location of the abnormal heartbeats. There are 2 broad categories of arrhythmias: those causing extra or rapid heartbeats (tachycardia), and those causing missed or slow heartbeats (bradycardia). Resting heart rates above 100 beats per minute (bpm) are considered rapid, and those below 60 bpm are considered slow. Both types of arrhythmias can cause the heart to pump inefficiently, leading to reduced blood flow to the brain and breathlessness because less blood is pumped to the lungs for oxygenation. As outlined above, the heart's electrical system must initiate, propagate, and recharge during each heartbeat. Deficiencies in this process lead to arrhythmias.

Ventricular tachycardia is a fast, regular beating of the heart caused by impulses originating downstream from the bundle of His or in the ventricles, or both. You may have heard doctors in television shows talk about the urgency of dealing with a patient's "V-tach." The heart rate may reach 280 bpm. Scars or structural damage within the ventricles are risk factors for developing ventricular tachycardia (Figure 5). Unsustained ventricular tachycardia may last no more than half a minute and is generally not life-threatening; however, sustained ventricular tachycardia is a harbinger of ventricular fibrillation, a life-threatening condition. About 90% of the 300,000 sudden cardiac deaths that occur in the U.S. each year are due to this arrhythmia (Mayo, 2002). The heart quivers uselessly without pumping blood, and this leads to the brain being deprived of blood, and unconsciousness within a few seconds. Without immediate medical attention, death results in a few minutes. The most effective treatment is defibrillation, a strong electrical shock to the heart. Many institutions where I live and work now have AED (automated external defibrillator) machines that can easily be used by laypersons to restart a fibrillating heart. Because of Alex's death, his college campus has been equipped with many AEDs.

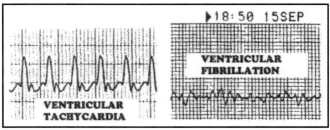

Figure 5. An ECG showing examples of ventricular tachycardia (VT) and ventricular fibrillation (VF). The VF is from my son's medical record after his fatal collapse on September 15, 2002

An important arrhythmia that is a risk factor for ventricular fibrillation is the long QT syndrome (LQTS). This arrhythmia is discussed in some detail in the September 2001 issue of the *Mayo Clinic Health Letter* information for laypersons and in a review article for cardiologists (Khan, 2002). This syndrome may have a genetic origin (ionic receptors in the heart cell membranes are abnormal, see Figure 2, page 4) or it may be caused by any one of a number of acquired conditions. Roughly 1 in 5,000 people are born with a genetic predisposition to LQTS. About 40% of these people never have problems; however, others will faint, often during exercise. Sudden cardiac death may occur in up to 10% of those with genetic LQTS. Acquired LQTS may be caused by administration of therapeutic drugs or electrolyte imbalances, specifically low blood potassium, magnesium, or calcium. As more drugs are discovered that can dangerously prolong the QT interval, this phenomenon has become an important research topic. I received a flyer that announced the 4th Annual Forum on Cardiac Safety and QT Prolongation in New Drug Products, to be held February 9-10, 2005 in Philadelphia, and I presume it was also sent to many cardiologists. Some of the more than 50 drugs that can prolong the QT interval do so by depleting potassium. QT prolongation by drugs is an important area of knowledge for cardiologists to be aware of to help them manage risk to the lives of their patients.

Tool 10: When ventricles fail to receive and respond to normal electrical impulses (Figure 1) they can beat on their own, leading to life-threatening arrhythmias. This is more likely to occur when the heart has pre-existing structural damage. A prolonged QT interval increases the risk of ventricular fibrillation.

How long does a QT interval need to be before it is "prolonged?" Cardiologists answer this by taking the measured QT interval from the ECG and correcting it using the Bazett equation, which has been used since the 1920s (Mirvis and Goldberger, 2001), or the ECG software prints the raw QT interval and the corrected value of QT on the ECG and labels them QT/QTc. The upper limit of a normal QTc for males can be found in any modern cardiology textbook. It is typically 440-450 milliseconds (Tadros et al., 2002; Olgin and Zipes, 2001; Mirvis and Goldberger, 2001; Myerberg and Castellanos, 1997; Richardson et al., 1998; Chou and Knilans, 1996).

Tool 11. A corrected QT interval above 450 milliseconds (ms) is abnormally long and this is an arrhythmia associated with SCD.

Bradycardia (slow heartbeat) is often associated with excellent physical fitness; however, it can also be an indicator of heart disease. Elite athletes often have heart rates below 40 bpm. Even as a 50-something-year-old runner, I had a heart rate in the low 40s. One arrhythmia that can seriously reduce the amount of blood the heart pumps by slowing the heart rate is called "sick sinus." This can be caused by an inherent pacing problem in the sinoatrial node itself (Figure 1, page 2) or by an impulse block that slows conduction or blocks it near the node. Conduction blocks may also occur in several places along the conducting pathway from the sinoatrial node to the ventricles. These can be partial blocks or complete blocks. Some of these blocks do not cause any symptoms.

Risk Factors for Heart Disease and Sudden Cardiac Death

Risk factors in medicine are specifically identified clinical or lifestyle findings that physicians use to establish whether a patient is likely to succumb to some disease. Risk factors can be divided into those that can be managed and those that cannot be managed. For the most part genetic risks cannot be eliminated, although medical advances are beginning to allow informed physicians to help patients overcome some of these previously unmanageable risks.

Assuming you and your doctor are aware of each controllable risk, you can choose to manage those risks or ignore them. In a clinical setting your physician should be looking for risk factors, such as high cholesterol, cardiac arrhythmias, or clinical symptoms (such as angina) that increase your risk of a heart attack or sudden cardiac death. Any physician who fails to identify risk factors is practicing uninformed medicine, and once the factors have been identified it is irresponsible for the physician to fail to inform the patient of the need to manage such factors. Furthermore, it is irresponsible medical practice to fail to put the management plan in writing so the patient can understand the risk. It must be emphasized that risk factors are not deterministic. People can carry high risks for heart disease for years and never have any overt heart disease. On the other hand, people with few if any known risk factors can suffer from idiopathic (cause unknown) heart disease.

Tool 12: It is the physician's responsibility to identify the risk factors present in clinical data and in the patient's lifestyle, and then guide the patient in managing them. This is called evidence-based practice (based on scientific evidence) of preventive medicine, and medical standards require that written instructions be provided to a patient who needs lifestyle risk management. You will find that you, holding this simple tool, would have been far more capable of helping my son live than his cardiologists ever were.

Risk and Informed Consent

Risk also has a key role in the informed consent process when your cardiologist proposes an invasive procedure. Are the risks of performing the invasive procedure clearly less than the risks associated with not knowing the information to be gained by the procedure? Can the same information be obtained by less risky methods? The answer to these questions is at the core of the physician-patient relationship.

Unfortunately, current practices of obtaining informed consent do not allow the patient to evaluate the true risk of a proposed procedure. Informed consent forms I have seen may list the potential adverse outcomes of a procedure, but no information is given to allow the patient to know what the probability of each bad outcome might be. Furthermore, physicians typically do not provide the patient with a list of alternatives to an invasive procedure and the pros and cons of each alternative. The physician believes he knows what is best for the patient, and expects the patient will follow his advice.

Tool 13: Genuine informed consent is the right of every patient. The basic elements of informed consent as defined by the AMA are as follows: The physician doing the invasive procedure should do the disclosures. Disclosures include informing the patient of the diagnosis, the purpose of the invasive procedure, the risks and benefits of the procedure, the alternatives to the procedure, and the consequences of not performing the procedure.

Chapter 2
Anatomy of an Adverse Event: Death of a Young Runner

Fitness and Running

My 17-year-old son became an avid runner in the fall of 2000 when he started college in a distant city. He had seen me run for several years in Houston, and without any encouragement, he decided that this was a sport at which he wanted to excel. From his days of competitive swimming he knew the dedicated effort it takes to become good at an endurance sport. In the spring of 2001 we ran our first races (a 5K and a one-mile run) together in Seabrook, Texas. Both races were part of the Pelican Run, named for the birds that gather in the waterfront park where the races begin and end. Both courses wind through woods and along a small bayou, then turn around and come back to the start. The trail consists of crushed granite. In the 5K race Alex and I ran together until about the 4.5-kilometer mark. At that point I kicked up our pace and asked him how much he had left for the finish. As I got ahead of him I heard a tripping noise behind me and turned around to see that my son had taken a nasty fall. I ran back to him to discover that his shoelace had caused him to trip and a large area on one leg and a smaller area on one hand were bleeding where his skin had been shredded. He got up, retied his shoe, and finished the race, winning his age group. He got the bleeding controlled in time to compete in the 1-miler. Two young guys who had not run the 5 K entered the miler and beat him, so he only took 3rd place in his age group. I had not seen this competitive side of my son for many years. I was proud that he was getting in shape and that he had the determination to recover from a bloody and painful fall.

My son and I ran several races together, and it was not long before he was easily beating his old man. The picture on the cover of this book shows him near the finish of one of the more brutal 5K races in the Clear Lake (Houston) area. The race is difficult because it is the first race of the year when the runners can count on extreme heat being a factor, and there is no shade on the course. I was proud that hot summer day in 2001 when Alex beat me in the Summer Kick-off Fun Run. This is a race in memory of James Glenn, a kicker for Texas A&M University who died suddenly of heart disease. His father conducts this race each year in honor of his fallen son and to earn money to give away as college scholarships.

After the awful events of September 2001 in New York City and Washington, D.C., Alex decided to serve his country by joining the Air Force Reserve Officer Training Corps. He continued running and decided that he was going to "max" the officer's physical fitness test. In the spring of 2002 he trained hard and when he was taken to Dallas in March for a routine military physical, the doctor discovered that he had a low heart rate (39 bpm) and administered an ECG, which he took to be normal for a trained athlete. Alex had a friend named Mike who was also in the Corps. It was a struggle for Mike to do well enough to qualify in the physical fitness test, let alone "max" it. One day in the spring when the cadets were being tested, my son put all he had into the test and nearly "maxed" it. He noticed that Mike was struggling with his running, so he ran back to Mike and then ran in with him, giving him encouragement and pushing him to give his all. Mike just qualified in physical fitness. Alex told me that he felt that his heart was going to burst from his chest as he pushed Mike toward the finish line.

In the summer of 2002 Alex went to Air Force summer camp at Ellsworth Air Force Base in South Dakota (Exhibit 1 page 17). It was a stressful time for him as his fragmented journal and his few allowed phone calls home testify. He told me that because of the heat and demanding physical stress, each cadet was required to drink 1-2 liters of water each time they exercised in the heat. Again he pushed himself to max the physical fitness test, but fell short by a few seconds in the 2-mile run. His journal from his time in summer camp reveals his physical and emotional struggles and his love of family, especially his little sister. It also provides a glimpse of his dreams, which he never had a chance to realize.

"We had our second physical fitness test today, and I improved 45 points from a 427 to 472. I am going to go for it [500 points] on the next test...I'm not going to get the base liberty this Sunday. I already missed my little sister's high school graduation, and now I'm not going to get to call her on her 18th birthday, which happens to be Sunday. Oh well, service before self, even though family has nothing to do with self. High school graduations and 18th birthdays occur only once in a lifetime, and it really sucks that I am going to miss it. I have decided that this [Air Force separation] is not for me. I want to have a family and settle down in one place for a while, but oh well. I feel as though I owe my country some service, and that is what I am going to give them...Tomorrow is Sunday and I am going to try to go to church to hopefully gather some inner peace, and lower my stress level...I am somewhat concerned about my calves; they have been painful for the last couple of days, and they don't seem to be getting any better; hopefully they will feel better in the morning...I

am disappointed that I didn't have 20 more seconds in me on my run this morning. Oh well, I'll have to work at it and max it at my DET [last fitness testing].

When he came back to Houston in early July, Alex continued running, and we ran the Lunar Rendezvous 5K race together later that month. This was to be our last race together, and also the last race for either of us. He beat me easily in the summer heat and humidity that only Houston and the Gulf Coast can produce in July. I can remember him waiting for me at the finish line and calling to me *"Good race dad."* Neither of us imagined that he would be dead in 2 months.

I Knew So Little about Hearts

From the end of "My Longest Drive" (Prologue), which took place after Alex's fatal collapse on September 15, I will now step back in time a few weeks earlier to the day when I was called in Houston and told that Alex had collapsed and recovered while running on the Jogging Trail at his university. This was Monday, August 19, 2002 (Exhibit 1). The trail is a loop about 2 ½ miles long and he was nearing completion of his second loop when he felt extremely weak, bent over, and the next thing he knew he was coming to in the ambulance. Suddenly, my healthy, athletic son had hit a hard bump in life, and I was called to go to an unfamiliar city and help him and his doctors manage his illness. After his collapse, which physicians call syncope, he was taken to a local hospital (Hospital 1). The cardiologists at that hospital rightfully insisted that he be admitted for further evaluation. He had become a cardiology patient.

Since no one in my immediate family had experienced serious heart problems, I knew little about how the heart functions and what can cause a sudden collapse. From my days working as a clinical chemist at the University of Maryland Hospital while I attended graduate school in the late '70s, I knew that potassium was important to normal cardiac performance. More recently, in my middle years, the federal agency I work for had offered to give me a laminated card with a tiny copy of my routine ECG so that if I were to have a sudden heart problem far from home, a record of my baseline ECG would be readily available. I had accepted their offer, and after trimming the rough edges and excess lamination, had found a place for this little card in my tattered wallet.

March 20	ECG performed by Air Force physician. No PVCs; QTc = 380 ms
Late May	Alex started Air Force summer camp at Ellsworth AFB, South Dakota
Early July	Summer camp ended for Alex; he returned to Houston.
July 20	Alex ran the Lunar Rendezvous 5K race in Houston with me.
HOSPITAL 1	
August 19	Alex collapsed (syncope) ~ 2300 while running at his university, but recovered spontaneously; he was taken to Hospital 1 by ambulance.
	2350 – Hospital 1 first ECG (occasional PVCs, QTc = 480 ms); serum electrolyte panel was completed.
	Medical record states that X-ray showed a "slightly globular heart."
August 20	0700 – Second ECG (no PVCs, QTc = 390 ms); serum electrolyte panel was completed.
	AM – Echocardiogram completed, results were supposedly normal.
	Austin cardiologist was asked to consult. He outlined plan for exercise stress testing, cardiac MRI, and then left heart catheterization and electrophysiology test only if necessary.
August 21	0622 – Alex's heart rate dropped to 28 bpm during his sleep.
	AM – Exercise stress test; Alex completed 21-minute Bruce Protocol.
	1120 – Serum magnesium requested for the first time.
	Cardiac MRI supposedly performed. Record shows "cancelled undiagnostic."
	"Family raised ? of neuron consult" noted in record by older cardiologist.
August 22	0940 – "Informed consent" obtained for left heart catheterization.
	1250 – Left heart catheterization done by older cardiologist.
	1607 – Cardiac monitor documentation showed multiform PVCs. This was the only one of 18 records by nursing service, starting from 1300 on 22 August, to show any PVCs.
	~1900 – Alex was discharged after a painful hematoma developed on his groin.
	Discharge report from Hospital 1 was written by a PIT.
	"Will discuss need for neuro consult with team" noted in record.

Exhibit 1. Timeline of Alex's cardiology events and medical testing in 2002 (continued on next page).

HOSPITAL 2	
August 23	Electrophysiology test at hospital 2. The medical record shows that a loop monitor was recommended, along with no running for now, and genetic testing for LQTS. Record notes frequent ectopic activity (PVCs).
CLINIC VISIT AND LETTER	
August 28	1315 – Hospital follow-up visit with physician in training at city clinic. The record of Alex's visit states that a pacemaker and an electroencephalogram were recommended by cardiologists and refused by Alex and/or his parents.
August 28	Letter sent from electrophysiologist to older cardiologist recommending that Alex have a loop monitor inserted and have genetic testing for LQTS (no mention of running ban).
HOSPITAL 1	
September 15	Evening – Fatal collapse while running at the university; CPR was administered, his heart was restarted by EMTs, and he was taken by ambulance to Hospital 1.
	~2200 – I was called in Houston and told my son was in deep coma with poor prognosis.
September 18	2230 – Alex died in Hospital 1. Heart sent to a pathologist in Dallas for autopsy.
December	Autopsy report received by my lawyer. Heart showed acute lesions in papillary muscles and left ventricular septum, and focal lesions on the external surface of ventricles. Older cardiologist called my wife in Houston to say Alex did not have a genetic disease, based on the pathologist's report.

Exhibit 1. Timeline of Alex's cardiology events and medical testing in 2002 (continued).

Was Potassium Replenishment Required to Save Alex?

Potassium is an element essential for life; it is carefully controlled by the body's physiological mechanisms. *As I described earlier, normal cardiac function depends directly on the availability of potassium, and responsible cardiologists pay careful attention to serum levels.* Some months after my son died I had a look at the hospital's website for patients to better understand the purpose of an ECG. That site lists 6 purposes for this testing. The 4th purpose is to show heart rhythm problems (arrhythmias) and the 5th purpose is to show changes in the electrical activity of the heart caused by an electrolyte imbalance in the body. *If my son's cardiologists had been cognizant of even these basic purposes for an ECG after he collapsed, they might have saved his life.* Please take out your Tool 4 that established that hypokalemia can cause a patient to have arrhythmias, especially acquired LQTS and PVCs. Let's sharpen it a bit. The "sharpening" question is: how low does a heart patient's potassium have to be before an informed cardiologist replenishes it in the patient?

Guideline medical standards for potassium replacement were published in the September 11, 2000 issue of *Archives of Internal Medicine* (Cohn et al., 2000). This journal is one of the journals published by the American Medical Association, and as such is highly respected. In 2002, the year of my son's death, the journal claimed more than 98,400 subscribers in at least 82 countries. The cost of this journal at that time was only $175 per year for an individual print subscription and $140 per year for an online-only subscription; both subscriptions could be purchased for just $185 per year. ***This journal is an inexpensive source of patient-care knowledge.***

The article presenting guideline medical standards for potassium replacement was based on a symposium held by the National Council on Potassium in Clinical Practice, which included seven physicians (mostly cardiologists and internists) from major medical centers and one doctor of pharmacology. ***The introductory paragraph of the article states: "it has been long established that the maintenance of normal serum potassium is essential in reducing the risk of life-threatening cardiac arrhythmias."*** From elsewhere in the introduction: "Normal serum potassium levels are considered to lie roughly between 3.6 and 5.0 mmol/L. The loss of just 1% (35 mmol) of total body potassium content would seriously disturb the delicate balance between intracellular and extracellular potassium and would result in profound physiological changes." In another part of the article the authors comment as follows: "Overt hypokalemia [low serum potassium] may be diagnosed when the serum potassium is less than 3.6 mmol/L...mild to moderate hypokalemia can increase the likelihood of cardiac arrhythmias in patients who have cardiac ischemia, heart failure, or left ventricular hypertrophy...The effects of hypokalemia on [ventricular] repolarization are magnified in many [cardiac] disease states." The process of repolarization is readily evident in a person's electrocardiogram as the T wave (Figure 3, page 5).

The cardiologists and internists conclude their guideline report for potassium replacement with *explicit* criteria for administration of potassium. For patients with cardiac arrhythmias they state the following: "Maintenance of optimal potassium levels (at least 4.0 mmol/L) is critical in these patients and routine potassium monitoring is obligatory. Patients with heart disease are often susceptible to life-threatening ventricular arrhythmias... The co administration of magnesium should be considered to facilitate the cellular uptake of potassium" The authors give no requirement to produce a specific diagnosis before beginning potassium replacement.

This is your Tool 4s (sharpened). According to the medical guideline, all the informed clinician needs to do is observe cardiac arrhythmias, such as PVCs or LQTS, and note that the patient's serum potassium is below 4.0 mmol/L to implement potassium replacement and monitoring of potassium in the serum.

You should examine Alex's ECG (Exhibit 2) with the medical guideline (Tool 4s) and Tool 11 in mind and determine if you would have implemented this standard. The emergency room (ER) physician, without knowledge of the ECG findings, suspected the possibility of an electrolyte imbalance as a cause of syncope and decided to have fluids (not containing any potassium) administered to him. The medical record also noted that he ran about 5 miles per day. I would not have expected an ER physician to be aware of this medical treatment standard that is your Tool 4s; however, the medical record shows that the cardiologists saw the PVCs and prolonged QT interval in Alex's initial ECG, and by that time Alex's potassium level was available for their inspection. You know that exercise in a hot climate leads to potassium depletion (Tool 5).

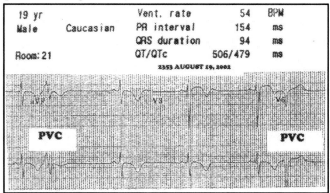

19 yr		Vent. rate	54	BPM
Male	Caucasian	PR interval	154	ms
		QRS duration	94	ms
Room: 21		QT/QTc	506/479	ms

1353 AUGUST 19, 2002

Exhibit 2. Parts of Alex's ECG, showing that he had a prolonged QT interval and PVCs on August 19 soon after he had syncope.

Once I had been told that Alex's potassium level was only 3.4 mmol/L, I asked a nurse what the normal range for this electrolyte was and she said it was 3.5 to 4.5 mmol/L. I asked her if they (meaning those treating my son) were going to do anything to increase that value. She said that they were going to do something. Alex's medical charts and the record from the hospital pharmacy, which I obtained much later, show that he was never given any medication with potassium in it. What would you have done if you were Alex's cardiologist?

A) Done nothing and waited to see what happened next.
B) Waited for the results of further testing.
C) Given potassium to Alex to get his potassium above 4.0 mmol/L.
D) Administered potassium to Alex, monitored his serum potassium levels, and immediately ordered a magnesium measurement.

Alex's cardiologists basically took action B. They ordered another ECG for the morning of August 20, another blood test, and an echocardiogram. It was not until after Alex's exercise stress test on August 21 that anyone thought to order a magnesium measurement. If you chose answer D using Tool 6, then you are already well ahead of my son's cardiologists.

Alex's older, lead cardiologist told me that he had concerns about my son's PVCs and his long QT interval, which when corrected for heart rate was about 480 ms (Exhibit 2). When he presented this information to me, I discounted the importance of the PVCs, saying that I knew that I had had PVCs after my exercise stress test. What I did not know was that PVCs are worrisome in a resting ECG in a patient who has just experienced syncope, especially during exercise. At that time I also mentioned to this older cardiologist my concerns about Alex's relatively low serum potassium after his syncope. ***That cardiologist told me that Alex's potassium was not sufficiently low to be concerned about.*** I also mentioned to this older cardiologist that I could get a previous ECG that had been done by the Air Force only a few months before. ***He told me not to bother getting Alex's previous ECG for now.*** Since I carried my little laminated ECG in my wallet, I was surprised at his disinterest in Alex's earlier ECG. At this point I began to doubt whether we should trust this older cardiologist with my son's care, but I could not think of an alternative. Alex had just returned to college to practice with the marching band. Classes had not started, so it was time to chill with friends, check out new girls, and tell stories of summer adventures. He would not want to come back to Houston for evaluation, and this older cardiologist had asked a consulting cardiologist from Austin to assist on the case, so I assumed that we would be getting a second opinion on the cause of Alex's syncope. ***At this point (August 20), two cardiologists were directly involved in my son's care, and so I believed that his life was in capable hands.***

Can You Make the Diagnosis?

Physicians have used ECGs as a tool for diagnosis of heart problems for many decades. The standard method for performing an ECG specifies placement of 12 electrodes on the skin, 6 near the heart and 6 at more peripheral locations on the body. The electrical impulses reaching these electrodes are recorded with sophisticated equipment so that the magnitude and timing of the beginning and end of the impulses can be measured to within a few milliseconds (one thousandth of a second). Software is sometimes used to analyze the shapes and durations of the impulses to derive a number of parameters (Figure 3, page 5). One of the most important calculated parameters is the time interval between the start of the Q impulse and the end of the T wave. The Q impulse marks the beginning of the QRS complex, which traces the ventricular depolarization as the muscular ventricles of the heart are stimulated to contract and push blood throughout the body. Depolarization is marked by the movement of potassium ions through the membranes of heart muscle cells. There is a baseline interval between the end of the S impulse and the beginning of the T wave. Finally, the T wave signifies repolarization, which involves, among other things, the movement of potassium ions through the membranes of heart muscle cells (Figure 2, page 4). The software applied to my son's ECG determined the average QT interval and then corrected that interval for his heart rate, giving the QTc value (Exhibit 2). *A prolonged corrected QT interval on the ECG is the basis for a diagnosis of LQTS as the cause of syncope* (Kruyer et al., 2002; Calkins and Zipes, 2001).

There are 2 general types of LQTS: genetic and acquired. The genetic form of the disease occurs because the ion channels that permit movement of ions in and out of the heart muscle cells are defective (Figure 2, page 4). The defects slow the movement of ions and cause an increase in the length of QTc because repolarization of the heart muscle cells is delayed. The other form of the disease is acquired as a result of a number of conditions including electrolyte imbalances and administration of certain drugs. *Hypokalemia is one of the most widely recognized causes of acquired LQTS* (Olgin and Zipes, 2001). Prolongation of the QTc interval is also caused by many drugs, some of which exert their effect by causing loss of potassium from the body. This phenomenon is so important that entire medical conferences are devoted to the subject of acquired long QT syndrome. *Even in my field of toxicology, the dangers associated with prolongation of QTc intervals have been recently recognized (Society of Toxicology, 2005).*

Since the diagnosis of LQTS is made from the QTc on the ECG printout, the only questions to be asked by the cardiologist are simple: what is the normal range for QTc, how long is the patient's QTc interval, and has the patient had this length of QTc all along (genetic form) or has the condition of a long QTc been acquired? A combination of the two causes is possible, but that is not relevant here. *My son's QTc interval after his initial syncope episode was 479 ms (in the August 19 ECG, Exhibit 2, marked as confirmed by a colleague of the older cardiologist) and told to me to be 480 ms by the older cardiologist. The consulting cardiologist wrote in the medical record that my son's QTc was ~ 490 ms.* Can you use Tool 11 to make the diagnosis? Here are your choices:

A) I choose to ignore the cardiology textbooks and Tool 11, so even though I know Alex's QTc is 480-490 ms, I will not make a diagnosis.
B) I will change the data to show that Alex never had a QTc of 480 ms, so there will be no diagnosis at this time.
C) This seems too simple to me, so I will not make a diagnosis.
D) Because Alex's corrected QT interval of 480-490 ms was well above the upper limit of normal of 440-450 ms, I think he had long QT syndrome.

Later you will be surprised to see which of the cardiologists chose A and B. If you chose option C, then you may want to sharpen Tool 11 to make the diagnosis of LQTS more certain; allow me to hand that sharper tool to you: the "Schwartz Criteria" for diagnosis of long QT syndrome. Schwartz and his colleagues established a point system in the mid-1980s and refined it in the early 1990s (Schwartz et al., 1993). About 9 months before Alex died, an article appeared in the "Curriculum in Cardiology" section of the *American Heart Journal* entitled "Long QT syndrome: diagnosis and management" (Khan, 2002). In that article the Schwartz diagnostic criteria were reiterated. The journal editors describe articles in the "Curriculum in Cardiology" section as *"Concise, comprehensive, contemporary articles presenting core, updated information __necessary__ for the continuing medical education of the modern clinical cardiologist"* (emphasis mine). You can use Exhibit 3 to determine your level of confidence in the diagnosis of LQTS in Alex's case.

You should be able to add up the appropriate point total to diagnose Alex's condition. Remember that Alex had collapsed (syncope) while running (a stressor), he had a low heart rate, and his QTc was ~480 ms. If you calculated a number that exceeds the 4 for a high probability of this diagnosis, then your Tool 11 has been sharpened and you can choose option D above with more confidence. You should notice that there are no absolutes here, only probabilities of a diagnosis.

	Points to give	Points for Alex
Clinical history		
Syncope		
With stress	2	____
Without stress	1	____
ECG findings		
QTc		
~480 ms	3	____
460-470 ms	2	____
~450 ms	1	____
Low heart rate	½	____
TOTAL FOR ALEX		____
Diagnostic scoring for LQTS: < 1 point = low probability, 2-3 points = intermediate probability, > 4 points = high probability.		

Exhibit 3. Application of the Schwartz criteria for diagnosis of LQTS in Alex's case.

Putting my son's clinical history of syncope with stress (2 points) together with the QTc of 480 ms from his ECG on August 19 (3 points), it was more than highly likely that my son had long QT syndrome. The remaining question is whether that syndrome was genetic or acquired. The way to determine this is to look at Alex's QTc intervals in several ECGs to determine how consistently it had been long. Table 1 (below) shows the dates of my son's resting ECGs and the resulting QTc intervals.

Date in 2002/ Time	QTc (ms)	PVCs	QTd (ms)	Serum Potassium	Source
March 20 AM	382	No	48	Not determined	Air Force
August 19 2350	479[a,b]	Occasional	120	3.4 mmol/L	Hospital 1, immediately after syncope
August 20 0730	390[b]	None	40	3.9 mmol/L	Hospital 1
Aug 20/1300 to Aug 22/2200	360-430	None	Not appl.	Not determined	17 hospital 5-lead ECGs[c]
August 23 noon	387	Frequent	Not det.	Not determined	Hospital 2, before EP test

Abnormal values are in bold letters. QTd is the dispersion (related to the range) of QT values. [a]This is the software-derived value; the consultant cardiologist estimated 490 ms and my calculation gave 485 ms. Technically the units are ms$^{1/2}$ when corrected for heart rate, but most simply use "ms" as the unit. [b]These values were confirmed by a colleague of the older cardiologist and printed directly on his ECGs. [c]I calculated the QTc values from QT and heart rate values written in the medical record by the nursing staff. These range in value because the measurements are difficult to do with the same accuracy as the 12-lead ECGs. One ECG after his left heart catheterization showed PVCs (see Exhibit 8).

Table 1. Selected values from Alex's ECGs showing abnormal values (occassional PVCs and long QT) and their disappearance when potassium normalized. The cause of the frequent PVCs will be discussed later.

You can make several possible diagnoses at this point:

A) The data are insufficient to make a diagnosis.
B) Alex may have the genetic form of long QT syndrome.
C) Alex had the acquired form of LQTS, but I do not know how he acquired it.
D) Alex had the acquired form of LQTS and I do know how he got it.

You will be amazed to see which cardiologists chose A or B as an option. For example, note in the August 28 entry in Exhibit 1 that Alex's cardiologists supposed that choice B was correct. They wanted to test him for the genetic form of the disease. However, even the most superficial inspection of the QTc values from this table shows that the value on August 19 was much greater than the others. If Alex had had the genetic form of LQTS, his QTc values would have been consistently high and they were not. This means that the form of LQTS that Alex had at the time of his collapse was the acquired form. Even without the ECG from the Air Force, which I had offered to obtain for the older cardiologist, by August 21 it should have been clear to an informed cardiologist that my son had the acquired form of the disease. Then a final question emerges: How did he acquire this disease and can it be treated? Did you already choose answer D?

The changes in Alex's serum potassium levels immediately suggest the cause of his acquired LQTS: hypokalemia (Tool 4). Reduced serum potassium is a widely known cause of acquired LQTS. The overnight administration (August 20) of saline by the ER physician may have indirectly improved his potassium level from overt hypokalemia to low normal. Knowing the mechanism of this is not essential. Perhaps the increase in his potassium was due to normal daily variations. Citing articles from 1998 and 1991, a review written by 6 physicians posted in July 2002 notes that there is a peak to trough variation in plasma potassium of about 0.6 mmol/L (Sica et al., 2002). The lowest values occur at night, which is roughly the time of day when Alex experienced his syncope episode. You should be asking, "How do you know that such a seemingly small increase in potassium (0.5 mmol/L) can reduce the QTc by 90 ms?" Be patient, you shall have your answer later when an "informed" cardiologist evaluates Alex's records.

Another feature of an ECG can suggest potassium depletion. *If hypokalemia is affecting an ECG, then the T wave is reduced in size, or if it is already negative, then it becomes a larger negative* (Sica et al., 2002). My son's baseline T wave was negative (at least in the V4 tracing), which is not too unusual for athletes. The negative T waves in his V4 tracings from four 12-lead ECGs (Exhibit 4) show the dramatic negative movement of this wave in one of his ECGs. I ask you to determine which of these ECG tracings suggests potassium depletion. *By polling neighborhood children ages 9 to 14, I determined that even a child can pick out the T wave that doesn't match the other 4, so I presume you can easily do that. You can draw your own conclusions as to whether this is sufficient evidence of potassium depletion in my son. Since Alex was a determined athlete, you should also recall Tool 5.*

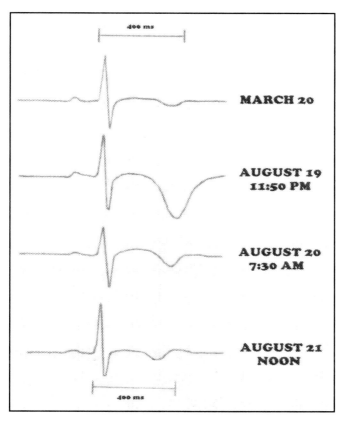

Exhibit 4. A comparison of the V4 tracings from Alex's ECGs.

Further evidence of the obvious cause of my son's deep negative T wave came from an unexpected source. As I was searching for drawings of the heart that would help me create my own figures for this book, I consulted a large, olive-colored text book on the heart illustrated by the physician Frank Netter and edited by another physician, Fred Yonkman (1969). Medical students for many decades have consulted these amazing books to learn anatomy and pathology. The volume on the heart contained the superb illustrations I expected to find, but it also had some examples of ECGs. As I scanned these tracings one caught my eye on page 70. It showed a large negative T wave in the V4 tracing, similar to my son's. Next to this was a figure of a more normal ECG. Allow me to paraphrase the story behind these 2 ECGs: An 18-year old school boy collapsed while running and was taken to a nearby emergency room. His initial ECG showed large negative T waves, so after keeping him for a month, the hospital discharged him with instructions not to participate in sports. A year later a better-informed medical center suspected the actual cause of the young man's inverted T waves and gave him oral potassium, which righted the T waves as shown in his second ECG. The comparison to my son's case is startling, except that Alex's physicians erred on the side of recklessness rather than conservatism, and they totally missed his need for potassium. This evidence is by no means definitive, but it is from nearly 40 years ago. Alex's cardiologists should have at least suspected potassium depletion as a cause of his deeply negative T waves and his collapse while running.

So why didn't his cardiologists make this connection to potassium? The answer is that they never looked at Alex's second ECG. I know they never looked for 3 reasons: the older cardiologist discussed Alex's long QT of 480 ms with me on the second day of his evaluation, but never mentioned that it had normalized to 390 ms as his potassium increased to 3.9 mmol/L; on August 23 this same older cardiologist and the electrophysiologist recommended genetic testing for long-QT syndrome, showing their ignorance of this change; and there is absolutely no mention of the ECG taken on August 20 in any of the medical records. It was simply a floating piece of paper. I had to look at the billing information from my insurance company, and then demand that the hospital send me a copy of specific ECGs, including the one from the 19th. This ECG and the one from August 20 were marked "confirmed" by a cardiologist who participates in the same cardiology practice as the older cardiologist.

The Dispersion of QT Intervals

You may have noticed in Table 1 that a new parameter has been entered in the column beside the QTc values; this is the dispersion in QT intervals. This parameter was mysterious to me for some time after Alex's death. As I did literature searches on QT intervals many reports involved discussion of the dispersion in a person's QT intervals. Soon I was able to deduce that this is the range of QT intervals in a subgroup of or all of the tracings on a 12-lead ECG. To my knowledge, in 2002 it was normally not computed by software applied to analyze ECGs. However, I found it easy to calculate this parameter from copy-machine enlargements of Alex's ECGs. I consistently used the V1 to V6 tracings in each of his ECGs since these were the clearest.

Large values of QTd had been understood as a risk factor for sudden cardiac death (SCD) at least a decade before Alex's death (Day et al., 1990). Although in 2002 cardiologists were not 100% in agreement, the association between a large QTd and SCD had been made in cardiology *textbooks* well before Alex's death (Castellanos et al., 2001). Many articles citing the association between QTd and SCD in infarct patients were published in the mid-1990s. Four of these are cited in an article entitled

"Sudden death due to cardiac arrhythmias," published in the *New England Journal of Medicine* (Huikuri et al., 2001). Normal ranges for QTd vary from about 50 to 65 ms (Mirvis and Goldberger, 2001; Perkiomaki et al., 1997; Castellanos et al., 2001). *Alex's QTd of 120 ms was so large that even by visual inspection of his ECG this should have been suspected.*

The meaning of a large dispersion in QT intervals is very important and some recent studies suggest that this parameter may be more important than the QTc in predicting the risk of SCD. If the patient's QTd is large, this means that some parts of the heart muscle are not repolarizing as efficiently as other parts. You can surmise that such a condition destabilizes the heart muscle because it is not functioning as a cohesive unit, thus inviting more dangerous arrhythmias to develop.

Tool 14: Dispersion of QT values above 70 ms is abnormal and associated with increased risk of SCD.

Alex's large QTd value was a 3rd arrhythmia present in his ECG from August 19. Having Tool 14 and knowing Alex's QTd values probably places you ahead of what an informed cardiologist in 2002 would have had in his tool box. On the other hand, at that time many cardiologists understood that a large QTd was a risk factor for SCD. Once I had the enlarged copies of the ECGs, the calculation of QTd required no more than 10 minutes per ECG. This is not much time to spend when a young man's life is at stake.

The Missing Magnesium

If you chose option D in the first set of answers (page 21), then you would have been ahead of Alex's cardiologists. The cardiologist who administered Alex's exercise stress test on August 21 observed during that test that Alex was a profuse sweater. My son was able to maximize the test; that is he was able to keep up with the treadmill for the entire 21 minutes of the test. Few people can do this. His profuse sweating prompted this cardiologist to request a serum magnesium level on my son. He stated to me that he wished that my son's doctors had been wise enough to ask for a magnesium level when he was first admitted after his syncope. Unfortunately, this cardiologist was unaware that clinical laboratories where serum chemistries are done are required, if they are certified by the American College of Pathology, to retain each sample for 1 week after it reaches the laboratory. This cardiologist could have asked the clinical laboratory to retrieve the sample from the late evening of August 19 and analyze it for magnesium. *Again, my son had encountered a cardiologist who was dangerously uninformed about the medical system within which he worked; he did not know that the clinical laboratory saves specimens for 1 week.* In defense of this cardiologist, he at least had the insight to order a magnesium level after the exercise stress test, which is a much more informed action than his colleagues had taken. My straw poll of a few other physicians working in hospitals revealed that most did not know that clinical laboratories save serum specimens for a week.

When I asked for the result of the magnesium determination done after Alex's exercise stress test, it was reported to me as normal. That is not a false statement; however, it is not the whole truth. His medical records, which I did not see until after his death, show that his magnesium level was 1.8 mmol/L, which is *extreme low* normal. Using your Tools 6, 7, and 8, you know that **hypomagnesemia often accompanies hypokalemia, and both conditions are associated with an increased incidence of PVCs, which are the gateway to SCD** (Myerburg et al., 1989). A patient with a low normal value of magnesium can be magnesium deficient (Sica et al., 2002). It is possible that a well-informed cardiologist would have thoughtfully evaluated my son's magnesium measurement, and then looked in more depth at his potassium measurements and his ECGs. Apparently, all the cardiologists were too uninformed and too busy to do this. *Thus another opportunity to correctly diagnose and treat my son was lost, and he moved another step closer to his death.*

The Mysterious, Missing Cardiac MRI and Uninformed Consent

The consulting cardiologist from Austin recommended that my son be given a cardiac MRI. Quoting the consultant's entry in Alex's medical record, "This [cardiac MRI] can sometimes give fiber orientation, estimate cardiac mass to exclude hypertrophic cardiomyopathy and finally detect the presence of arrhythmogenic right ventricular dysplasia. On occasion it is also possible to determine the course of the coronary arteries. If the coronary arteries cannot be identified during the procedure, then I would recommend left heart catheterization." This is consistent with what we were told at the time. Clearly, the goal of Alex's cardiac MRI was to learn enough about my son's heart so that he did not have to undergo cardiac catheterization, with which are associated a risk of injury and a risk of death from about 1 in 130 to 1 in 700 depending on the study population (Davidson and Bonow, 2001).

The cardiac MRI was not a pleasant experience for my son because he had been thoroughly hydrated via his intravenous (IV) line and halfway through the process he had to urinate. Another man, who was known to my son, had to help him urinate without disturbing the ongoing capture of MRI images. I recall that when he returned to his hospital room, he was upset at this necessity during the MRI, but at least he had remained still and completed the procedure. The nurse who brought him back complimented him on how well he tolerated the procedure. He had done his part, but as you are about to see, others had not done theirs.

I refer to my son's MRI as mysterious because my insurance company was never sent a bill from the hospital, nor did his medical record contain any radiologist's report. For many months my lawyer had forbidden me from contacting the hospital, so I could not inquire as to its outcome. I asked him to look into this, but he never did. When I no longer needed this lawyer's services, I called the hospital and was told that my son's MRI was cancelled. I told them that that was bull. Finally, they faxed me a record showing that it was "cancelled undiagnostic." As I was to find out later, that's hospital-speak for "we screwed up."

Eventually, I was to discover that Hospital 1 had just received a software upgrade on their cardiac MRI machine and my son was the first patient on which the use of the new software was attempted. Unfortunately, the operators present at the time had not been fully trained in use of the new software, so the cardiac MRI was incomplete or aborted, depending on which description I choose to report. *I have been told by an expert that the cardiac MRI as it was performed on my son had no chance of accomplishing any of the goals expressed by the consulting cardiologist from Austin.* However, I was also told that Alex's cardiac MRI could have been repeated at the Hospital 1 and done properly because persons with the appropriate skill were available. In addition, routine cardiac MRIs were performed in a nearby hospital in Dallas.

You have your Tool 13 on informed consent; however, you might be interested in exactly how cardiologists have defined the specific situation for which a left heart catheterization is contemplated. In June 2001 the *Journal of the American College of Cardiology* published an article defining informed consent (Bashore et al., 2001). In section VII of that article, the ethical concerns associated with keeping physicians centered on the patient's best interests are described. Using their words, "Changing practice patterns in medicine, including the expansion of both managed care and for-profit physician entrepreneurial ventures have altered the relationships among physicians, patients, and payers, creating potential conflicts of interest for the physician in maintaining the patient's best interest." *Thus, according to this guideline, "physicians must provide accurate and unbiased information about the patient's medical condition, disclose alternative choices and potential conflicts of interest, and obtain informed consent, delineating the potential risks and benefits (and alternatives) of the diagnostic and therapeutic strategy."* Initially, my son's cardiologists did a reasonable job of following this medical standard. They recommended performing a cardiac MRI, and if this did not show certain features, then a cardiac catheterization and electrophysiology test would be in order. Our son's assumption, and ours as his parents, was that a competent cardiac MRI could be done at Hospital 1.

I ask you to get hold of Tool 13 or use the cardiologist's specific definition of informed consent. Imagine that it is time for you, as his cardiologist, to inform Alex about left heart catheterization. This procedure poses a small risk of death and many other complications, but you want to receive his consent for the procedure to be done. Which of the options below would you have selected?

A) Even though I know the cardiac MRI was not done right, I will simply tell Alex that the cardiac MRI did not show what we hoped, so he needs to undergo a left heart catheterization to rule out "life-threatening" conditions. I'll tell him a scary story to help him make the right choice.

B) Admit to Alex that mistakes were made in his first cardiac MRI and that better-trained staff is now available and we would like to repeat the test here. This may enable him to avoid invasive testing, but he can choose to go straight to the invasive testing if he wants.

C) Tell Alex that cardiac MRIs are routinely done at a hospital in Dallas, and we can make arrangements to have the test done there.

D) Tell Alex he has a choice of either of options B or C.

Of all the emotionally painful discoveries I have made about my son's medical care, the discovery that Alex's cardiologists chose option A ranks second only to the false statements that his doctors placed in his medical records. *It is one thing to be ignorant of standards and too busy to take a thorough look at the medical test results, but it is quite another to deliberately withhold key information from a frightened young man and his frightened parents so that he can be cajoled into signing informed consent papers for invasive, revenue-generating testing. The medical record shows that the older cardiologist had given orders to get the "permit for cath." It did not say inform the patient of his options.*

How does the cardiologist who made choice 'A' sell an invasive test to a frightened 19-year-old boy worried about the list of bad outcomes that could be caused by the procedure? Once the physician has circumvented the informed consent process (not told the patient his actual choices), he simply uses fear mongering to counter the patient's fear of a bad outcome from a left heart catheterization. Specifically, in Alex's case we were told the woeful story of basketball star Pete Maravich, who died suddenly during a pick-up basketball game when he was 40 years old. An autopsy showed that Maravich had no left main coronary artery and had widespread patches of dead heart muscle (Van Camp and Choi, 1988 in Rowland, 1999). The older cardiologist's stated goal of the catheterization was to rule out the possibility that Alex had anomalous (abnormal) coronary arteries. Information I obtained much later showed that the older cardiologist was doing catheterizations at a rate of about 450 procedures per year. Clearly, this invasive procedure was a major source of revenue for this physician and he was a good salesman. *It was not in his interest either to inform us of the efficacy of non-invasive testing such as a cardiac MRI, which had been known for several years (McConnell et al., 1995; Post et al., 1995), or to tell us that the hospital's attempted cardiac MRI was aborted.*

You might ask if a left heart catheterization was even indicated in this situation. Citing articles from a few years earlier, Eckart et al. (2004), in their article entitled "Sudden death in young adults: a 25-year review of autopsies in military recruits" recommend that "screening for anomalous coronary arteries with imaging techniques (echocardiography, computed tomography, or MRI) be strongly considered in any young patient initiating an exercise program who presents with symptoms that may be referable to cardiovascular disease." The possibility of using catheterization to screen for disease is not even mentioned by these authors. The justification for doing a catheterization in my son's case was marginal at best, but the sales job was superb.

I will describe Alex's catheterization shortly. After having the catheterization and eventually recovering, he was discharged from Hospital 1, and the next morning he went with me to Hospital 2 for an electrophysiology test. First, you should look at his discharge summary.

The Error-Laden Discharge Summary from Hospital 1

Alex's cardiologists had failed to apply the guideline for potassium replacement when the patient has arrhythmias, they had failed to diagnose acquired LQTS, and they had missed the implications of his borderline low magnesium; however, there was a 4th and final opportunity for my son's cardiologists to piece together the puzzle of his illness. But they were in a hurry and dumped the task of completing the hospital discharge summary on a physician in training (PIT). The discharge summary should have been done by Alex's attending physician. This man was board certified in family medicine and had considerable knowledge of cardiology because his wife had had some heart problems. We met with this attending physician several times during the course of my son's evaluation and trusted his judgment. But the task of writing my son's discharge summary was assigned to a PIT who, to my knowledge, had never seen him as a patient. Her discharge report, presumably written on the day of his discharge (August 22) is little more than an assortment of errors and oversights. This might not be surprising given that her medical education was secured in a Third World country and she was "in training."

In her discharge summary one set of laboratory data (from August 19) is listed, but there is no mention of my son's second set of laboratory data from the morning of August 20, nor of his borderline low magnesium measurement from August 21. She states, "ECG shows sinus bradycardia with occasional PVCs," as if my son had had only one ECG. There is no mention of the prolonged QTc interval of 479 ms or the inverted T-waves in his first ECG, nor does she mention that the PVCs and long QTc had disappeared in my son's second ECG taken on August 20. In the section entitled "HOSPITAL COURSE" she states, "The patient was evaluated by Electrophysiology." *In fact, my son's electrophysiology test was not done until August 23 at Hospital 2, one day after she supposedly wrote his discharge report.*

A second peculiar statement appears: "The patient might get a work up for a possible seizure disorder as an outpatient in Houston, including neuro evaluation and Electroencephalogram." This statement seems to be an embellishment of a note made in the record by the older cardiologist: "Family has raised ? of neuro consult & EEG." In fact we had asked the family practice physician whether my son was given over to the cardiologists before his need for a neurological evaluation was considered, and that physician gave us a long explanation of why the cause of my son's syncope was not neurological. The cardiologists never recommended any sort of neurological evaluation or electroencephalogram. In addition, the PIT's discharge report makes no mention of my son's missing cardiac MRI, which was recommended by the consultant cardiologist and supposedly performed on the morning of August 21. In the 2½ pages of the discharge report, this neophyte physician had overlooked critical results in my son's medical records and couldn't even copy statements in the records correctly for the purpose of his hospital discharge report.

A 4th and final chance to properly diagnose and treat my son was lost because the responsibility for preparing Alex's discharge summary was delegated to an incredibly careless and inexperienced physician.

The Invasive Procedures: Worthless and Painful

After his aborted cardiac MRI, my son had two invasive procedures to evaluate the condition of his heart. The first of these was a catheterization, which involved insertion of a wire and a catheter (tiny plastic tube) into his femoral artery accessed in his groin after it had been punctured under local anesthesia. The catheter was guided along a wire that had been pushed into the left side of his heart, and then pressure measurements and a ventriculogram using dye were made. The catheter was moved to the coronary arteries and more dye was injected to allow visualization of these arteries. I was permitted in the "control room" and observed the images of the dye flowing through his arteries. The entire procedure required about 10 minutes; however, Alex's recovery from the procedure was to be prolonged.

He was taken from the catheterization laboratory to a hospital bed and remained there for several hours while I sat with him. He had heavy weights on his right groin to prevent the entry wound from breaking open. *I do not recall the exact circumstances, only that something happened and he suddenly had a large hematoma on his groin.* This is not the kind of hematoma one receives from giving blood, it was a 3-dimensional bleb caused by the artery breaking open under his skin. Later he likened the pain to a knife piercing his groin. He started groaning, *"Oh God, oh God, get help, I need help."* I ran to the nurse's station and got her to come down to his room as quickly as possible. He was in extreme agony until the nurse at last repacked his wound. His stay in the room was extended for at least 2 hours. For the first time in his life my son had experienced an invasive medical procedure; he would experience only one more before his fatal collapse in 3 weeks. The attending family physician had told us that the electrophysiology (EP) test, which was to be given the next day, would be less painful because it involved insertion into veins rather than arteries. This prediction turned out not to be true.

The next day I checked my son into a second hospital in town for his EP test, which was administered by a colleague of the consultant cardiologist from Austin. This time I was excluded from observing the procedure. I was forced to wait in the hall for a time twice as long as the time told to me. The procedure that was done to Alex included insertion of catheters into veins in both sides of his groin, and then pushing them up through his veins until they reached his right ventricle. I can recall being extremely worried that something untoward had happened to him. I was relieved to at last be allowed in the room where the testing was done and to see that Alex, who was still lying on the gurney, appeared to be fine.

The electrophysiologist told us, with the older cardiologist present, that Alex should consider having a loop monitor inserted in case he collapsed again. A loop monitor is a device that is inserted under the skin and records heartbeats of the wearer when the wearer activates it. We were told that Alex could activate its recording capability if he started to feel faint. *We were told that he needed to avoid vigorous activity (such as running) for now, and that he should have genetic testing for LQTS by Dr. Jeffrey Towbin in Houston, which the electrophysiologist offered to arrange.* The electrophysiologist talked about defects in receptors that cause the genetic form of long QT syndrome, and he mentioned potassium receptors. *Once again I mentioned my concerns about Alex's hypokalemia, but the electrophysiologist did not respond.*

At this point I was concerned because absolutely no treatment was being proposed to Alex, and so there was no reason not to expect him to collapse again. So I asked what the course of action would be if he were to collapse again, and I was told by the older cardiologist that he would need to consider a pacemaker or an implantable cardioverter-defibrillator (ICD). A pacemaker is an implanted device that has wires reaching into the right side of the heart through which it stimulates the heart to beat, and an ICD is an implantable device that can shock a fibrillating heart to resume normal rhythm. I knew an ICD would not be acceptable to the military, so I asked if a pacemaker would put him out of the Air Force. The older cardiologist told me that it would. Alex had expressed disgust with his IV line, so I asked if he would have to have an IV for insertion of the loop monitor and was told that it was legally required, but that the monitor could be inserted under his skin in only 10 minutes in the older cardiologist's office. I asked if a Holter monitor (a strapped-on device with battery pack and electrodes for sensing heartbeats) wouldn't be sufficient and was told by the older cardiologist that it would not be; *Alex needed a loop monitor, according to the older cardiologist and the electrophysiologist.*

My son said very little as he lay on the gurney during the discussions. He seemed reasonably attentive to me, but as I was able to deduce much later, he probably did not remember any of this discussion. Here are the drugs he was given and the times they were injected into his blood stream: Versed (1 milligram) at 1233 and again at 1410, and Fentanyl (50 micrograms) at 1411. The record shows that the electrophysiologist discussed his 3 recommendations with Alex and me between 1411 and 1423. The sedative dose of Versed alone in adults should not exceed 2.5 mg and the full effects of the drug are usually present in about 3 minutes after administration. The purpose of giving the drug is sedation, relief of anxiety, and amnesia. *Amnesia! It is very likely that the electrophysiologist's administration of these drugs caused my son to forget much if not all of what was told to him.*

I went with Alex as he was wheeled to a hospital room and then gently lifted from the gurney and lowered onto the bed, the orderlies being careful to keep the packing on his new wounds in place. He was a distraught young man. He told me that the cardiologists had given him so much drug that his heart was pounding so hard that the table he was on was shaking. In addition, he told me that the electrophysiology procedure was much more painful than the catheterization.

The Unwritten Advice

Alex's doctors had told him and me 3 things while he was sedated on the gurney after his EP test: he needed to have a loop monitor inserted, he needed to avoid vigorous exercise for now, and he needed to have genetic testing for LQTS. *I remember trying to reassure him that I was certain he did not have a genetic disease.* He felt that he was in excellent health, he had endured the endless weeks of Air Force officer's basic training earlier in the summer, and now he might have a genetic disease!

I tried to make small talk with my son as we "watched" a TV near the far corner of the room. *Alex's demeanor was like what I would expect from a human who had been severely abused. He had a far-off look in his eyes, he would not talk to any extent, and he was very hungry.* I tried to comfort my son, but he would not be comforted. How could he have a genetic disease? What had been the point of all the painful testing he had endured?

His somber mood was broken when a medic showed up with a catheter to insert into his bladder. Rather than accept the insertion, he was told that he could get up and urinate. *When he did this one of his groin wounds opened and he bled profusely into the toilet and on the floor as he hobbled back to his bed.* His bleeding wound was quickly repacked, and the catheter was forgotten for the time being. A woman from housekeeping came and scrubbed up my son's blood, which had poured freely down his leg and had been freely spread over the floor.

After several more hours the nurse indicated that Alex could be released. He was given a sheet of instructions. *The only restriction on the sheet was that he was not to drive for 24 hours. There was nothing about his need for a loop monitor, the ban on running for now, nor the genetic testing. This is a failure to use Tool 11, which requires that needed management of risk factors be put in writing for the patient.*

I ask you to form an opinion of the importance of putting the ban on running in writing to him.

A) A doctor should have to tell his patient only once, even if the patient is only 19 years old and sedated, that he should not run "for now." He should have remembered. It is not our responsibility to write down everything for the patient.

B) The fact that Alex was running when he experienced syncope and then later when he died does not mean that the ban on running mattered. Even if we cardiologists did not write this down for him, it did not matter.

C) It was a catastrophic mistake not to put the ban on running in writing for Alex, especially since the next physician he saw (the PIT) was never told to reinforce this recommendation and Alex probably was unable to remember the verbal recommendations because of the drugs that were in his system when he was informed of the recommendations.

Our Decision against a Loop Monitor

My son and I left the hospital with me driving his old Blazer that he had bought from his grandpa a few years before (remember, he was not to drive). We drove over to a Mexican restaurant on Valley Mills Road and got some real Mexican food and a headlamp and radiator hose for his Blazer. Over dinner we discussed the pros and cons of a loop monitor. It did not make sense to us to have it inserted, since it would have to be activated to record, which would be nearly impossible for a fainting person to do. We decided that he would tell the physician he was to see the following Wednesday, August 28, that he did not want the loop monitor. I had assumed that this office visit was with a cardiologist. I was wrong. My son's care had been passed off to a PIT and we were not told this. I do not know if this is a violation of any medical standard, but if it is not, then it ought to be. Perhaps I should have asked, but I never imagined that Alex's care would be placed in the hands of someone in training in another medical field.

The Botched Hospital Follow-up Visit with the PIT

On August 28, 2002, my son saw the last physician he would ever see. She worked at a clinic in town and had written his hospital discharge summary. Remember the PIT! I have already pointed out her sloppy hospital summary, and that quality of work was to continue in the write-up of Alex's office visit. Here are some statements from her records and my comments (refer to Exhibits 5 and 6):

PIT: "He [Alex] was advised by [the older cardiologist] that he needs a pacemaker, but since he wants to join the Air Force, he does not want the pacemaker because it would prevent him from joining the Air Force. His heart rate during hospitalization was between 40 and 60."

A

RECOMMENDATIONS:

1. **Implantation of a loop recorder device** to assess for the possibility of rhythm disturbance should any recurrent syncopal episodes occur.

2. Withhold vigorous activity for now.

3. Refer to Dr. Jeff Towbin regarding genetic testing for long QT syndrome at Texas Children's Hospital in Houston

----

B

  This letter will summarize my findings on Alex James, who you will recall is a very pleasant 19-year-old gentleman who recently had a syncopal episode with exertion. He was initially seen by [the older cardiologist] who recommended comprehensive electrophysiology study. He was found to have borderline prolongation of the QT interval.

  On August 23, 2002, Alex underwent comprehensive electrophysiology study at [Hospital 2] in [town]. He was found to have no inducible supraventricular or ventricular tachycardia. The QT interval shortened appropriately with isoproterenol infusion; however, the longest corrected Q-T interval during the course of the study was found to be approximately 490 ms, which is mildly abnormal. **We discussed options going forward, and the decision was made to recommend a loop recorder for Alex**, along with referral to Dr. Jeff Tobin in Houston at Children's Hospital, who has significant research experience with long Q-T syndrome. I certainly think it would be worthwhile to proceed with genetic screening to determine whether Alex has one of the known mutations for long Q-T.

  This is certainly a difficult case. I do not think that Alex currently requires ICD implantation. He has had a single episode, and we do not know that he has long Q-T syndrome, nor that his event was arrhythmic in etiology. I think that a loop recorder will be helpful, certainly should he have any recurrent symptomatic episodes.

Exhibit 5. The recommendations told to Alex at Hospital 2 after his EP test (A) and part of the letter from the electrophysiologist to the older cardiologist (B).
Note that the recommendation against vigorous activity was omitted from the letter, and there is no mention in either of a pacemaker or electroencephalogram.

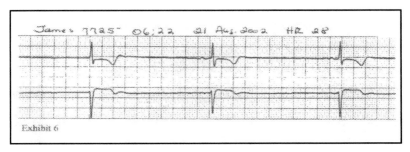

Exhibit 6

Exhibit 6. Heart rate of 28 bpm.

Comment: The statement about the older cardiologist saying that Alex needs a pacemaker is false. The medical record from Hospital 2 and a follow-up letter (dated August 28, 2002) from the electrophysiologist to the older cardiologist clearly show that the only device recommended to my son was a loop monitor (Exhibit 5), which he decided to decline. His heart rate during hospitalization was in fact as low as 28 bpm (Exhibit 6); the record shows that. That rate is well outside the range stated by the PIT, and it is important that it was actually that low. Since the loop monitor recommendation was never given to Alex in writing, it is possible that he told the PIT that he was refusing a pacemaker; however, this seems unlikely in view of the next statement about his heart rate being between 40 and 60. Alex knew very well that his heart rate had gone to 28 bpm one night in the hospital, and he was rather proud of this since he took this as an indication of excellent physical fitness.

PIT: "Patient had a work up done including echocardiogram, exercise stress test, and electrophysiological studies which were all normal."

Comment: This is a strange statement because Alex was also to have had a cardiac MRI and a left heart catheterization. Since the electrophysiology test showed frequent ectopic activity (PVCs), it was not normal. Perhaps the PIT had electrophysiology and echocardiography mixed up. Look at the results of Alex's echocardiogram to determine if any parameter was outside the normal range (Exhibit 7, next page).

PIT: "His EKG showed sinus bradycardia with some premature ventricular contractions. His chest X-ray was normal."

M-MODE (Adult Normal Values)	
RIGHT VENTRICLE (0.7-2.3 cm)	<no result>
SEPTAL WALL (0.8-1.1 cm)	0.73
LEFT VENTRICLE (D) (3.5-5.6 cm)	5.53
LEFT VENTRICLE (S)	4.07
LVPW	0.80
AORTIC ROOT (2.0-3.7 cm)	2.73
LEFT ATRIUM (1.9-4.0 cm)	3.53

**Exhibit 7: Results of Alex's echocardiogram on August 20 at Hospital 1.
Can you identify the measurement that was outside the adult normal range? Later it
may help you find a killer.**

Comment: Only two of Alex's many resting routine ECGs showed
PVCs. The ECG immediately after his syncope (Exhibit 2, page 20) and
the one a few hours after his left heart catheterization (Exhibit 8) were
the only ones to show PVCs. Sporadic PVCs were found in his continuous
monitoring records. Finally, the hand-written record and the PIT's hospital
discharge summary state that Alex's X-ray showed a "slightly globular
appearing" heart. This is not normal, or it would have been called normal
by the radiologist.

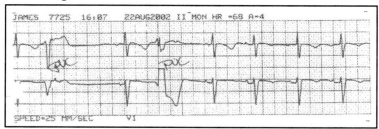

**Exhibit 8: Alex's ECG a few hours after his left heart catheterization. Note the pair
of PVCs.**

PIT: "An EEG (electroencephalogram) study was advised by cardiology,
but patient and parents refused it. They will consider it later on in Houston
as they live in there. Since patient and parents are refusing a pacemaker,
there is really nothing else we can offer him."

Comment: *These are both false statements. We (the patient and his
parents) were never offered an electroencephalogram by anyone. In fact
we were told by the attending family physician that Alex did not need
to have one. Would we refuse a non-invasive electroencephalogram,
and then allow invasive procedures that risked his life? We never said
anything about having an electroencephalogram done in Houston. As I*

41

wrote before, the statement about refusing a pacemaker is inconsistent with my son's medical records, and is patently false.

What is strangely missing from this office visit is any comment about Alex not engaging in "vigorous exercise" as he was verbally advised to do "for now" while sedated after the electrophysiology test. There is also no mention of the intention to do a genetic test as recommended after his EP test. There is no mention in the record that the PIT even asked Alex if the insertion wounds he received from his catheterization and EP testing were healing properly. I have often wondered if the PIT had any communication with the older cardiologist after the EP test on August 23. It seems that she did from her erroneous statement about the EP test, but why were the other key recommendations left out of the record or perverted from a loop monitor to a pacemaker?

I made my best effort to discover when this record of Alex's clinic visit was last modified. I did this through the clinic, through the Texas Medical Board, and through the Department of Health and Human Services, which supports the clinic. All of them were able to almost completely stonewall me from gaining definitive information. *The clinic record does show that the PIT "reviewed" my son's medical record on October 9, 2002, 3 weeks after he died. I have made several attempts to contact her through the clinic where she saw my son, but that clinic has refused to forward my questions to her.*

You should have a chance to express your perspective by choosing among the descriptions below (you can choose more than one option):

A) It was clear that Alex did not have any real heart problems. He maximized the exercise stress test, after all. Thus, his cardiologists made a reasonable choice in assigning his hospital summary and follow-up care to a physician in training. Besides that, cardiologists do not get paid much for doing this kind of simple follow-up work.

B) I totally trust physicians to write truthful statements in medical records. The accusations you are making must be wrong.

C) Hospitals are very busy places and it simply is not the fault of Alex's cardiologists that they assigned his hospital summary and follow up visit to a PIT. How could they have known how ill he actually was?

D) The PIT was simply a victim of circumstances and I would be pleased to have her treating my child.

E) The cardiologists had made about all the money they could through their testing and it did not show any big problems, so it was reasonable to hand off his care to an inexperienced physician.

F) Alex's cardiologists should have taken a cautious approach, ensuring that the hospital summary was done by an experienced physician, preferably a cardiologist, and that his hospital follow-up visit was with an experienced physician who was familiar with his hospital record.

The Good Guys

As I began to think about writing the story of my son's death and the role of cardiologists in it, I realized that I had found something wrong with almost every aspect of his "treatment." Nonetheless, I vowed to myself that I would identify those physicians who had done their job well and discuss their excellence. The first physician who did well, in my opinion, was the emergency room physician who examined Alex immediately after his non-fatal collapse. I think being an emergency room physician must be one of the most difficult jobs in the medical community. Suddenly, with little or no warning, a person can be delivered into your care with an immediately life-threatening illness or injury. Decisions must be made quickly and knowledgeably. Furthermore, this front-line doctor must know when to call in medical reinforcements to assist him. Alex's emergency room physician was wise enough to order an ECG after his admission to the hospital and he suspected an electrolyte imbalance, apparently based on Alex's history as a runner. Because he suspected Alex had an electrolyte imbalance, he ordered an electrolyte panel for the cardiologists to have the next morning. The data stemming from his decisions were precisely what the cardiologists needed the next morning to make evidence-based decisions: a potassium level of 3.4 mmol/L, an occasional PVC, and a QTc interval of 479 ms to diagnose LQTS and apply the medical guideline for potassium replacement. The emergency room physician had done his job well; he acquired the data needed for the cardiologists to make correct decisions. Such decisions were never made.

	2353 August 19	0736 August 20
Vent. Rate	54 BPM	52 BPM
PR interval	154 ms	152 ms
QRS duration	94 ms	92 ms
QT/QTc	506/479	420/390

19 August 2353	Sinus Bradycardia with occasional Premature ventricular complexes Left anterior fasicular block Probable Persistent juvinile T waves Possible Lateral infarct, age undetermined T wave abnormality, consider inferior ischemia T wave abnormality, consider anterior ischemia Abnormal ECG No previous ECGs available Signature on File
20 August 0736	Sinus bradycardia with 2nd degree SA block (Mobitz I) Septal infarct, age undetermined Possible lateral infarct (cited on or before 19-AUG-2002) Probable persistent juvenile T waves T wave abnormality, consider inferior ischemia Abnormal ECG When compared with ECG of 19-AUG-2002 23:53 Premature ventricular complexes are no longer Present Sinus rhythm is now with 2nd degree SA block (Mobitz I) Left anterior fascicular block is no longer Present Serial changes of Lateral infarct Present Signature on file

Exhibit 9. Comparison of Alex's ECGs from August 19 and 20.
Note that the cardiologist interpreting the first ECG was not made aware that I had offered to get Alex's ECG taken by the Air Force a few months earlier. These records clearly state that Alex's ECGs are abnormal, that his PVCs disappeared overnight, and that the QT/QTc interval shortened from quite abnormal to perfectly normal. A pathologist friend of mine has written to me his opinion that the "possible lateral infarcts" are probably associated with the subepicardial lesions (focal fibrosis) found by the Dallas pathologist in Alex's heart after he died (see Exhibit 10, page 67).

The second physician who, in my opinion, did his job very well was the cardiologist in the older cardiologist's practice group who interpreted Alex's ECGs from August 19 and August 20. This cardiologist apparently used state-of-the-art software to glean considerable information from the ECGs. In Exhibit 9 I have provided a copy of his descriptions of the findings in the 2 ECGs, including those that are quantitative. These medical records display the remarkable number of worrisome findings in the 2 ECGs and note the dramatic changes in just 8 hours. Many of the worrisome comments concerning Alex's ECGs are about phenomena that can be attributed to his athletic condition, but a prolonged QT/QTc cannot be dismissed that way, and the disappearance of the PVCs cannot. These ECGs were really the last piece of evidence the other cardiologists needed to get a correct diagnosis. Obviously, Alex's QTc was prolonged on the 19th, and obviously it reverted back to normal overnight. The diagnosis is obvious.

I believe a 3rd physician was highly responsible during Alex's initial evaluation after his syncope. This was the family practice physician who spent considerable time with my son discussing various facets of his case. This physician gave us an explanation of why Alex's syncope was cardiogenic and not neurogenic, and the subsequent medical findings testify to his insight. I am confident that if this experienced physician had written Alex's hospital discharge summary, he would have deduced the proper diagnosis of his illness. I think he probably was not aware of the guideline for potassium replacement established by the National Council on Potassium Replacement in Clinical Practice.

Alex's Last Run

Perhaps a week after his last doctor visit on August 28, 2002, Alex began easy runs on alternate days. For most of these runs he took along a friend to match his strides on the university trail. About two weeks after his last visit to a doctor, I asked Alex during one of our frequent telephone calls if he had experienced anything that would have caused him to activate a loop monitor if he had had one. He said no to answer my question. He said that he had felt tired while playing basketball, but that after a drink of water he was up and playing again. On the morning of his last day of life on earth, he called us while we were at church. The cell phone connection was so poor that we agreed that he would try to call us again in the late afternoon. On the hot evening of September 15, 2002, Alex decided to run the trail, but none of his friends could go along. I learned from students later that he was running swiftly as he passed them on the first part of the trail, and then they saw him collapsed and dying as they caught up to him in a few minutes. A former lifeguard happened by and gave Alex CPR. When the medics arrived, they had to shock his heart 3 times to restart it. My firstborn son officially died 3 days later in the hospital where he had received uninformed, unethical, and careless medical care only weeks before. The American health care system calls this an adverse event; for those of us who loved Alex or called him friend, this was a heart-breaking time as we watched his body slowly give up its last traces of life.

Chapter 3
A Futile Search for Justice

In Chapter 2 I shared with you the journey my son experienced in the "health care system" and the many ways his cardiologists should have recognized his compelling need for potassium replacement, communicated with him honestly to avoid invasive testing, and written down their recommendation not to run. My insight into these mistakes evolved over several years as I contacted more knowledgeable people and taught myself more cardiology. In this chapter you will be invited to apply more of your cardiology tools to understand the mindset behind opinions provided by several cardiologists who looked at Alex's medical records after he died. The purpose of their reviews was to determine if Alex's physicians had met standards of care during his evaluation. I hope that you have a strong opinion about that already and are prepared for some rather silly arguments from cardiologists.

When I began to recover from the anguish and grief I felt after my son's death, I realized that I needed to look at his hospital records to determine whether his brother and sister needed evaluation for the genetic form of LQTS. I was so hesitant to directly ask for his records that I persuaded a neurologist at my agency to request Alex's records from the hospital where he had died. In a week or so my colleague called me to say that the records had arrived. *When I looked at the ¼-inch-thick pile of papers, I quickly realized that I was up against some incredibly error-filled medical work. I blew my stack when I read the words of the PIT that my son and his parents had refused a pacemaker.* I knew my mind was not what it was before my son died, but I recalled clearly that Alex's cardiologists had recommended a loop monitor, and not a pacemaker. I recalled that we had discussed options if he had another syncope event. If that were to happen, *then* he would have to consider a pacemaker or implantable cardioverter-defibrillator (ICD) to protect his heart.

I also recalled that the older cardiologist had told me that Alex's corrected QT interval was about 480 ms; however, the one ECG that was sent to me showed that it was only 390 ms on August 20. I had to dig out my medical bills and see that my insurance company was billed for 3 ECGs, and so I requested the 2 unsent ECGs and everything else I could imagine in the record. *Even before I saw the ECG of August 19 showing a QTc of 479 ms, I was beginning to suspect that my son died of untreated acquired LQTS.*

In early October 2002, I decided to go to a lawyer. He told me that the small pile of medical records that were originally sent to me was not complete by any means. My lawyer also requested my son's records from both hospitals and from the clinic where the PIT worked. He warned me that I was unlikely to receive justice. He mentioned a tragic event that was unfolding at the time. As I recall, a 4-year-old girl had received a much publicized heart-lung transplant, but the hospital mismatched the tissue, so she died quickly after the transplant. My lawyer pointed out that her doctors were already asserting on TV that she was likely to die soon anyway, so what was the issue with a little tissue mismatch. *He said the typical physician mindset accommodates almost anything, but never an admission of a mistake.* Eventually I received more of my son's medical records and some on other patients as well (so much for their privacy!). No information came about the cardiac MRI that I knew my son had been "given," but for the moment I was satisfied.

I did economic battle with the second hospital and the Austin-based cardiologists who administered the electrophysiology test because they kept sending my dead son their bills despite my requests that they be sent to me and that I be sent a copy of his medical records. More than 4 months after Alex died these jerks were still sending bills in his name to his former home address. By early February 2003, I had begun to understand how seriously they had mishandled my son's case. I wrote letters to the Austin cardiology group and to the second hospital, telling them that I should not have to pay anything because of their errors. They both agreed that my insurance company's payments had been sufficient. The fee total to the electrophysiology doctor's practice from my insurance company was $11,500, and the total expected by the hospital was $13,400. Not bad for a couple of hours of work torturing a 19-year-old boy who would not even have needed to have the test performed if he had been properly diagnosed in the first place! *I was relieved when I finally got the second hospital's records of the electrophysiology testing and it showed clearly that my son was offered a loop monitor and not a pacemaker.* My memory was not lost after all, but my fight had only just begun.

One part of the fight that I lost was obtaining a clear copy of Alex's Air Force ECG from March 2002. The copy I was provided by the Air Force was partially unreadable, so I began calls and emails to obtain a clear copy of the original. After more than a dozen calls and emails to places spread across the country, I finally gave up any hope of getting a clearer copy of Alex's Air Force ECG. It seems that when airmen die, their medical records enter an inaccessible abyss. The copy I did have showed clear profiles and the numbers for his heart rate and QT were clear. The value for his QTc was unclear, so I ended up calculating it using a standard equation.

The Cardiologists Review the Records: The TV Cardiologist

December, 2002: The first cardiologist to perform a formal review of my son's medical records after he died was identified by my lawyer from a TV show in which the cardiologist presented himself well. His credentials as a cardiologist were beyond reproach and showed that he was board certified in 3 subspecialties by the American Board of Internal Medicine. He charged my lawyer $2,250 for a 3 ½-hour review of my son's records, and he was also gracious enough to address follow-up questions that I had without additional charge. All this occurred about 4 months after my son's death and I had not gained many of the tools that you now have, so my questions were not well taken.

After Alex's death, his heart had been sent to a pathologist in Dallas for autopsy. The pathologist had reported finding lesions in several places in Alex's heart, including "healing myocarditis" in the outside of the ventricular free wall (not the septum). I will discuss this report in detail in Chapter 4. The cardiologist concluded that Alex's care met standards and this heart injury was the cause of death. His observations could certainly be accepted if my son had suddenly died without any medical evaluation beforehand. For example, if someone dies suddenly of heart failure and myocarditis is found in the heart, then it is reasonable to take that as the probable cause of death because nothing else is known. This TV cardiologist, even though he *did* have access to extensive medical records, maintained the physician-protective position that myocarditis was all that mattered in my son's death. He was mistaken to do that.

The first mistake he made was to state, referring to Alex's ECG of August 19, 2002, "It was not known if the patient had a previous ECG, or if these abnormalities [seen in the 19 August ECG] were necessarily new." The TV cardiologist apparently overlooked the Air Force ECG from March 2002 that my lawyer had sent him (and that I had offered to get for the older cardiologist). That ECG clearly showed that the LQTS seen on the August 19 ECG was absent a few months earlier. Sandwiching the V4 tracing of the August 19 ECG between the one done in March and the one done 8 hours later on August 20 illustrates the remarkable difference in the negativity of the T wave and its prolongation at least 150 ms beyond the before-and-after ECGs (Exhibit 4, page 27). This alone is compelling evidence of an acquired condition at the time of syncope that had been reversed by something the next day.

The second error the TV cardiologist made was to sidestep the issue of diagnosis of acquired LQTS by asserting that my son's ECG on August 19 showed a range of QTc intervals from 440 to 480 ms. This is his crass attempt to take away your Tool 11 that you used to diagnose LQTS. The cardiologist confirming the ECG found an *average* QTc value of 479 ms, the older cardiologist told me that Alex's average QTc was about 480 ms, the consulting cardiologist estimated (in the medical record) Alex's average QTc at 490 ms, and my estimated average from his ECG was 485 ms. The V4 tracing on this ECG shows a huge negative T wave and a QT interval of 600 ms and, when this is adjusted for his heart rate of 54 bpm, yields a QTc of 569 ms in this single tracing. Obviously, 569 ms is not between 440 and 480 ms! The esteemed TV cardiologist seems to have miscalculated the range of the QTc values in my son's ECG. Furthermore, even if we used the TV cardiologist's numbers, Alex's diagnosis was in fact LQTS according to criteria published in the journal *Circulation* (Schwartz et al., 1993) and the *American Heart Journal* (Khan, 2002). If you did the calculation in Exhibit 3 (page 24) for diagnosis of LQTS using the ECG value of QTc, you should have gotten 5.5 points, exceeding the value of 4 needed for a high probability of this diagnosis. Even if you used a QTc value of 460 ms (halfway in the range proposed by the TV cardiologist), the point score would be 4.5. *This is a clearly missed diagnosis, not only by my son's cardiologists, but also by the triply-board-certified TV cardiologist who evaluated Alex's medical records. The TV cardiologist tried to steal your Tool 11s, but I trust that you held on to it.*

An obvious diagnosis of LQTS should have been made with high confidence. The TV cardiologist does state, "Alex's admission potassium level was mildly reduced (3.4 on 8/19/02), which could have accounted for his initial QTc interval prolongation, but would not have explained the other abnormalities seen in his ECG." As you know, it certainly would have explained the deep negative T-waves and the PVCs. Unfortunately, later in his report this doctor states, "The changes seen on his ECG were not sufficiently specific to make a diagnosis, and could be interpreted as suspicious for LQTS, or the ECG of a normal athletic heart." You, equipped with your Tools 11 and 4, know full well that this is pure bunk. *Reduced potassium levels are a well-known cause of acquired LQTS (Olgin and Zipes, 2001) and to assert that the diagnosis of acquired LQTS could not be confidently made from my son's ECG is ridiculous on the part of the TV cardiologist (see Table 1, page 25).*

This multi-boarded cardiologist also seemed to be totally unaware of the medical guideline for potassium replacement published in the Archives of Internal Medicine (Cohn et al., 2000). That guideline, which is your sharpened Tool 4, specifies that cardiac patients with arrhythmias and blood potassium below 4.0 mmol/L should receive potassium replacement. There was no need to specifically diagnose my son's anatomical heart condition or even his acquired LQTS. All the cardiologists had to do was to know and apply this medical guideline, set and published by a national expert panel to render effective treatment, which was potassium replacement.

I want to make two further comments about the view of electrolytes displayed in this esteemed cardiologist's analysis. He commented that my son's magnesium level (1.8) was normal, which is technically correct but incomplete. This value is *extreme low* normal and it is well known that an individual can be magnesium depleted and still have a low normal magnesium level. He also stated in reference to my son's second admission after his fatal collapse that "His (Alex's) admission laboratory tests showed a normal potassium." In fact, his admission potassium was 3.8 mmol/L, which is low normal, and the TV cardiologist's statement is true.

The rest of the story is that this sample was taken roughly an hour after my son's fatal collapse and in that hour many cells in his body died. This is proven by the release of enzymes, which are highly concentrated inside cells (your Tool 3), out into his blood. Potassium is also highly concentrated inside cells and as they died, copious amounts of potassium were released into his blood. Furthermore, even in the absence of cell death, hypoxia is known to cause movement of potassium from inside the tissue to the blood stream (Sica et al., 2002). The whole truth is that my son's potassium level at the time of his fatal collapse was most likely well below the value of 3.8 mmol/L measured when he had been delivered to Hospital 1.

Although the TV cardiologist made many other deductions that are biased in favor of the cardiologists who attempted to diagnose my son's illness, I will take issue with only 2 more. The TV cardiologist states, "A cardiac MRI can be useful in detecting some heart abnormalities, but it is limited in requiring that an abnormality be large enough to be seen. In addition, MRI is a new test, for which expertise in interpretation is still in the developing stage." The fact is that nearby in Dallas, cardiac MRIs were being done routinely and interpreted accurately by Dr. Ron Peshock of The University of Texas Southwestern Medical School. He frequently used gadolinium as an image enhancer, and this almost certainly would have allowed visualization of the lesions in my son's heart (Friedrich et al., 1998). *If a proper cardiac MRI was not available at the in-town hospital, then my son should have been offered the opportunity to be given a proper cardiac MRI by Dr. Peshock.*

Furthermore, was cardiac MRI such a new test as the TV cardiologist suggested? The AMA in 2002 listed 3 category-I current procedural terminologies for cardiac MRIs. Each of these is listed as "with or without contrast [media such as gadolinium]." One is called "cardiac MRI for function, with or without morphology, complete study." The expert panel that defines category-I current procedural terminologies requires the following: "1) Food and Drug Administration approval of the procedure, 2) that it [the procedure] be performed by many physicians/practitioners across the United States, and 3) that efficacy of the procedure is established and documented in the peer reviewed literature." The TV cardiologist did not know what he was talking about! *Cardiac MRIs were fully recognized by the AMA as effective procedures in 2002.* Of course, as the TV cardiologist asserts, "expertise in interpretation was still in developing stage in 2002," but expertise in interpretation of ECGs, which had been around for a century (Wellens and Gorgels, 2004), was also still developing in 2002. For example, I have a cardiologist friend who is working on a software package to automatically calculate QTd from ECGs, and a new T-wave alternans test from Cambridge Heart (Bartlett and Steels, 2006) has been given AMA approval as a current practice terminology diagnostic to supplement ECG interpretation. *I trust that you recognize the uninformed excuse-making that the TV cardiologist is engaged in here. He did note that the cardiac MRI supposedly done in Hospital 1 was missing from Alex's medical record.*

The TV cardiologist states near the end of his evaluation, "That no serious arrhythmias were found on Mr. James' initial evaluation, nor any evidence of a [structural] heart abnormality, left his physicians with the dilemma of having no specific problem to treat...Given that Mr. James fainted while exercising and had an abnormal ECG, he was appropriately evaluated thoroughly for heart and rhythm abnormalities, a search which turned up empty." The search for rhythm abnormalities turned up empty! You know better than this. Furthermore, the reality is that when Alex's potassium was low it momentarily unmasked the lesions in his heart, which I will show in Chapter 4 were not really myocarditis. An article about syncope in young athletes in the journal *The Physician and Sports Medicine* (Puffer et al., 2002) cautions in half-centimeter-high bold letters:

"Physicians must exercise care in evaluating deep T-wave inversions accompanied by symmetric T-wave contour... or prolonged QT interval; these patterns can indicate underlying pathology." I ask you to determine whether Alex's T-wave on August 19 was deeply negative and symmetric (Exhibit

4, page 27). We have already dealt with Alex's QT interval, showing that it was quite prolonged on August 19.

Myerburg and his associates have published extensively in medical journals and cardiology textbooks on the interaction of functional abnormalities such as hypokalemia and structural abnormalities such as ventricular fibrosis (Myerburg and Castellanos, 2001). Below I expand a diagram (from Figure 4, page 7) they have used to explain SCD; studying this diagram will allow you to sharpen your Tool 8.

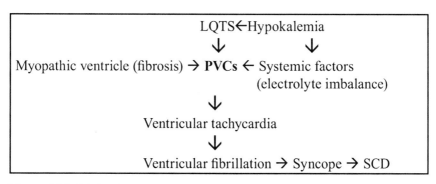

Figure 6. Model showing how sudden cardiac death (SCD) resulted in Alex's specific situation. Figure 7 (page 71) shows how additional factors came together to produce his SCD.

What Myerburg asserts in the peer-reviewed medical literature is crucial to understand. He states, ***"Structural cardiac abnormalities are commonly defined as the causative basis for SCD. However, functional alterations of the abnormal anatomic substrate usually are required to alter stability of the myocardium permitting a potentially fatal arrhythmia to be initiated."*** Note the pivotal role of PVCs. The truth is it took the ventricular lesions, the vigorous activity, *and* the hypokalemia to cause Alex to collapse. His hypokalemia was readily controllable and was at a level that, according to a widely published clinical practice guideline, required therapy. The disappearance of 3 arrhythmias in Alex's ECGs when his potassium went to 3.9 mmol/L confirms the importance of applying the potassium replacement guideline. When Alex's serum potassium increased to 3.9 mmol/L his PVCs, his long QT interval, his high dispersion of QT intervals, and his deep, symmetric T waves all disappeared—*temporarily.* ***You can decide if the TV cardiologist's opinion is tainted by bias, inattention to Alex's medical records, or simply being ignorant of diagnosis and treatment guidelines. The search was not empty as the TV cardiologist suggests. The only thing empty was the minds of the cardiologists.***

The Academic Cardiologist Reviews Alex's Records

By early March 2003 I had found another lawyer, who happened to also be a physician. During my first meeting with him in his office, he told me that the reason he went to law school after medical school was because he had witnessed so many acts of malpractice in medicine. He seemed to be the right person to aggressively pursue my allegations. This lawyer found a second cardiologist to review Alex's medical records. He was an academic cardiologist associated with a pediatric syncope clinic in Houston, and he asserted that my son received medical care that was adequate according to the standard of care. I was invited to discuss the case with this cardiologist, as long as I paid for his time myself. My second lawyer indicated in a letter to me that this academic cardiologist had determined that the software had misinterpreted my son's ECG from the 19th of August, and that Alex never had LQTS. This was despite the fact that a colleague of the older cardiologist had "confirmed" the results of my son's ECGs on the 19th and 20th. The academic cardiologist had determined this software error by his own hand calculation, asserting, "The computerized algorithm that includes the intervals that were created by Alex's QT and QTc intervals on that EKG relies on an algorithm that includes the intervals that were created by Alex' PVCs." This is another cardiologist attempting to steal your Tool 11 used to diagnose LQTS. *I went to visit this cardiologist with mixed feelings. On the one hand I knew that his opinion about the software misinterpretation was wrong because I had calculated the QT values by hand myself; on the other hand, I was seeking to listen, understand, and hopefully accept his opinion that my son's life could not have been saved, that Alex's cardiologists had done all they could reasonably be expected to do.*

Three topics stand out in my memory from our meeting, which must have lasted for 1½ hours. First, when I indicated that I had done the QT calculations by hand and had gotten results within a few milliseconds of the software's calculation, the academic cardiologist quickly dropped his opinion that my son never had LQTS. Second, after I presented him with what I felt was compelling evidence that Alex needed potassium replacement therapy based on the changes in his ECGs (I was not yet aware of the published clinical practice guideline for potassium replacement— your sharpened Tool 4), *he told me point blank that he would never have given potassium replacement in response to a serum potassium of 3.4 mmol/L. Apparently, I was not the only one in the room who was unaware of the medical standard for potassium replacement when arrhythmias are present.* Third, I went on to describe what I felt was compelling clinical evidence from the ECGs that there was some sort of pathology in my son's heart even though the catheterization and electrophysiology tests were more or less normal. I tried to convince this man that my son's doctors failed to take an informed and cautious approach to his diagnosis and treatment. His response was that the other side (the lawyers supporting the accused physicians) could line up a dozen cardiologists who would swear that it was "myocarditis" alone that killed my son, and that myocarditis is a challenge to diagnose in life. Here you see the cardiologist's mindset: if you cannot find a specific anatomical diagnosis, then you are not going to be held accountable, regardless of the evidence.

I recall leaving the room with a sense of relief that perhaps it was only the "myocarditis" itself and that my son's doctors had been sufficiently careful. By the time I got to my car, however, I was having second thoughts about this conclusion. The academic cardiologist never actually said that it *was* "myocarditis" that killed Alex, only that that is what the other side would claim. Despite his assertion about not treating a potassium level of 3.4 mmol/L, I was still convinced of its importance. Much later, with the help of a cardiologist colleague where I work, I found the medical standard for potassium replacement in the presence of arrhythmias and sent the reference from *Archives of Internal Medicine* (Cohn et al., 2000) to the academic cardiologist and to the TV cardiologist. I hope they will wake up to the importance of this critical electrolyte in normal cardiac function.

In a letter to me, my second lawyer reflected some of the opinions of the academic cardiologist. Here I will take issue with some of his opinions as stated in that letter, which I will assume is an accurate description of the academic cardiologist's opinions. One statement that reflects a limited knowledge of cardiology is this one: "As to the subendocardial lesions in his ventricular septum and papillary muscles, Dr. Academic agreed with the letter you received from Dr. Pathology. Those lesions were acute and were the result of Alex' cardiac arrest, not its cause. As to whether those lesions might have resulted from Alex' August 23 EP test, Dr. Academic pointed out that no object was introduced into Alex' left ventricle during that procedure. And any injury caused by his heart catheterization would have been limited to mere bruising and insufficient to cause either necrosis or ventricular fibrillation." ***The medical literature shows that a clumsy catheterization can do much more than simply bruise the heart.*** There are sporadic reports of more serious damage to the heart, and the website of the hospital where the catheterization was performed indicates that one of the possible injuries to the heart from catheterization is perforation of the heart (Brueck et al., 2004; Tamura et al., 1993; Marine et al., 2001). Furthermore, how does a cardiac arrest cause lesions specifically on the left side of the ventricular septum? *The academic cardiologist was feeding my physician-lawyer a biased story and the latter was accepting it.*

In another part of the lawyer's letter he asserts, "Dr. Academic pointed out that the gold standard of EP testing is the ability to induce ventricular tachycardia or ventricular fibrillation during the EP study." *That cardiologist's opinion overlooks the observation made by the electrophysiologist that Alex had frequent PVCs during the testing.* It also overlooks the contribution hypokalemia made to his syncope a few days before the testing. My son was not hypokalemic during the EP testing. Finally, and this is crucial, it overlooks the well-known possibility of false negatives (failure to identify a true arrhythmic cause of syncope) in the EP testing. Calkins and Zipes (2001) in a cardiology textbook chapter called "Hypotension and Syncope" cite an earlier publication (Krahn et al., 1995), asserting that "EP testing does not always identify the arrhythmic cause of syncope because transient abnormalities such as those caused by ischemia or fluctuations in autonomic tone may be missed." In my son's case the transient abnormality that had disappeared was hypokalemia. *Any cardiologist administering an expensive and invasive test like an EP study must know of the false negatives that the test can yield.* Apparently, the academic cardiologist was unaware of or unwilling to admit this fact.

One related statement I recall from the 3 days of dying that Alex's body underwent came from a colleague of the cardiologists in Austin. In reference to the EP testing, he asserted that "we were betrayed by our tests." I accepted that as a reasonable statement at the time; however, now I know it was a self-delusional perspective. Alex's cardiologists were not betrayed at all; they were simply ignorant of the limitations of their testing, and of course, they had already totally missed the diagnosis of acquired LQTS. The ones betrayed were my son and those who loved him. *The truth then is this: Alex and his family were betrayed by the uninformed and inattentive practice of cardiology by his physicians.*

By early October 2003, my second lawyer and I had parted ways. His work on Alex's case occurred during the time when tort reform was looming in the state of Texas. In my opinion, this lawyer took on too many cases hoping to identify the best ones to pursue before September 2003, when the door was nearly shut on accountability of physicians for their mistakes. Alex's case was not one of those he chose to pursue.

Because of the academic cardiologist's mistaken opinion on the length of Alex's QT interval, I began to suspect that cardiologists were not all that well informed in their technical discipline. Sporadic articles in the newspaper over the next few months suggested that this was true for many cardiologists. Another frightening family event reinforced my fears about the competency of cardiologists and internists.

Laura's Story

In the spring of 2004, 1½ years after Alex died, a physician at the clinic at Texas A&M University discovered that my 19-year-old daughter had a heart murmur. The physician detected this with a simple stethoscope and recommended that she have it evaluated at home. Laura finished out the semester and we obtained an appointment for her with an internist who worked in the same practice as my wife's internist.

Thinking "Once fooled, shame on you physicians; twice fooled, shame on me," I pulled out my trusty textbook on cardiovascular disease (Braunwald and Perloff, 2001) and read about heart murmurs. A heart murmur is a series of audible vibrations that produce a swooshing sound when it is listened to with a stethoscope. There are 3 major categories: systolic (occurring during heart contraction), diastolic (occurring when the heart is not contracting), and continuous (spanning portions of systole and diastole). Laura was told she had a systolic murmur. Systolic murmurs are further divided into those that occur in the early, middle, or late part of the systole. Murmurs are also characterized by their intensity according to a loudness scale that dates back to 1933. There are 6 grades of loudness: 1, heard only with special effort; 2, soft, but readily detected; and so on to 6, loud enough to be heard with the stethoscope just removed from the chest wall. There are many possible causes of a heart murmur, but identifying the 2 factors above (location in the cardiac cycle and loudness) leads to considerable focus toward the possible cause.

The internist listened to Laura's heart and proposed to do a series of blood tests and an ECG, and asked a cardiologist to do an echocardiogram. My daughter was found to be slightly anemic, but otherwise the blood and heart tests were deemed normal. For example, her ECG showed a QTc of 393 milliseconds. The information presented in the echocardiogram was confusing to me, so I asked for an appointment with the internist to discuss my daughter's results. I actually faxed my 6 questions ahead of my visit so that he would have a chance to review them and have an answer to them.

When my daughter and I arrived for the office visit, we found the doctor a little indignant at my asking so many questions. My first question was what type of systolic murmur my daughter had and what was its intensity. The internist's answer was that characterizing murmurs as I had read was a bit of a lost art and that physicians rely more on the ECG and echocardiograms to identify the cause of the murmur. He had not been able to characterize her murmur. We agreed that her ECG was entirely normal, but the internist was unable to interpret the echocardiogram results for me and suggested I get an appointment with the cardiologist. I asked for Laura's complete record to take to the cardiologist, and was given the internist's report. On the way to the cardiologist's office (just downstairs) I began to look at her records from the internist. I was shocked at how error-filled they were.

The internist had written in the history that Laura's brother "had a heart murmur, electrolyte problem and subsequently died while exercising." Under family history he wrote "The patient's brother is deceased. The cause of death was Healing mild Carditis; Atrial Fibrillation." Most disturbing of all was that under the "Cardiovascular" heading in reference to Laura he had written "Grade I/VI holosystolic murmur." It was clear that he was a very poor listener. We never said anything about Laura's brother having a murmur and it seems that the internist did not recognize "myocarditis" as a disease entity, writing instead "mild Carditis." Finally, I was puzzled how he had concluded that my daughter had a grade I, holosystolic murmur when he had clearly told us in his office that he had not been able to characterize it.

I spent an entire month trying to get in phone contact with the internist to ask which was true—what he had told us in his office or what his records showed. I found that the only way I could get a call back from his office was to call in on the "doctors'" line (I'm a Ph.D. doctor, after all!). To me this is one of the most irksome aspects of dealing with a physician. There is the pretense that they operate in circles we mere patients (or parents of patients) dare not penetrate. Somehow a doctor's call is always more important than a patient's call. This is an affirmation of the physician-centered practice of medicine in the United States.

At last I was able to speak with the internist on the phone and ask him which statement was true, what he had said or what he had written. He said that what he told us in his office was true. Then I asked him why he had written something else in Laura's medical record. He repeatedly refused to answer that question and only repeated that what he told us in his office was true. He told me I should not have been looking at her records anyway. Finally, he told me that if I thought I was so smart, why didn't I go out and buy an audiotape of murmurs and see if I could figure out the different classifications.

My daughter took the recommended vitamins and iron supplements for several months and her anemia and murmur became history. For me this was yet another example of a physician specialist engaged in careless and uninformed practice of medicine. No harm was done this time, but that does not excuse the nature of his practice of medicine. On September 18,

2005, three years after her older brother died, Laura completed a triathlon in San Antonio in honor of her fallen brother.

Now, I ask you to return to the evaluations of my deceased son's medical records.

The Disciplinary Process Review Committee (DPRC)'s 1ˢᵗ Secret Cardiologist

In March 2004 I submitted my allegations of wrongdoing by Alex's doctors to the Texas State Board of Medical Examiners (TSBME), now called the Texas Medical Board (TMB). The Board engaged 2 other cardiologists to examine my son's medical records; however, I have very little insight into the substance of their opinions because their thinking was kept secret from me. After an investigational period of 5 months (March to August, 2004) the TSBME investigator concluded that "the evidence does not indicate a violation of the Texas Medical Practice Act." Within 2 weeks I shot a long letter back to the TSBME investigator, with copies of it sent to my state representative and the Governor of Texas. I followed this with a letter indicating that I wanted to appeal the initial decision. Soon, I received a letter from the Director of the TSBME explaining that the secret cardiologist concluded that *"A thorough evaluation to exclude structural heart problems and arranging the early involvement of an electrophysiologist, resulted in the management of care that met the general standard in this situation. Because the extensive testing performed revealed no structural heart problems, the patient's primary cardiac disease could not have been identified."* I do not know if the secret cardiologist explained his opinion further, but if this statement is true, then it is an incredible whitewash of the situation. It assumes that effective treatment of my son's illness would have required a specific *structural* diagnosis. This is utter nonsense! *The cardiologist's opinion ignores the existence of the Guidelines for Potassium Replacement that are independent of any structural diagnosis, it ignores the missed diagnosis of acquired LQTS, it ignores the presence of 3 risk factors (PVCs, LQTS, and high QTd) for sudden cardiac death that were controllable, it ignores the strong suggestions in the ECGs of structural injury of some kind (Puffer, 2002), it ignores the fact that the tests administered are known to be unable to detect potentially life-threatening lesions, and it ignores the fact that my son was never given a written warning not to run.* This is to say nothing of the failure to give Alex enough information for him to give truly informed consent and the peculiar spread of false information by the older cardiologist and PIT that my son was offered and refused both a pacemaker and electroencephalogram.

On October 5, 2004, my appeal, which I was later told was the first one ever lodged, was accepted and I was allowed to present my opinions to the DPRC in writing and in person in February 2005. During my presentation, which had been distributed in writing to the members of this committee, I gained further insight into the evasive thinking of one cardiologist. This came when the cardiologist chairman of the DPRC engaged me in a discussion of my son's cardiac MRI, or lack thereof. I had raised the issue that my son could not have given informed consent because he was never told that his attempted cardiac MRI was aborted. Instead of addressing the issue of lack of informed consent, the chairman cardiologist went on and on about how a cardiac MRI would never have revealed all the information needed to eliminate the possibility of structural abnormalities in my son's coronary arteries that could have caused his syncope. *This is a classic trick of expert physician evasion: Ignore the real question, substitute a more convenient question, and then answer the dickens out of the convenient question.*

The DPRC's 2nd Secret Cardiologist

I have less insight into the conclusions of the 2nd secret cardiologist engaged to deal with my appeal. The chairman of the DPRC read a few parts of this cardiologist's conclusions to me. I think the one that is most disturbing is the expert's opinion that my son's cardiologists actually *exceeded* medical standards for his care. He also made some remarks about the lack of culpability of the cardiologist who had done the EP test. This is interesting because I had not made any allegations against him. To me this suggests that the 2nd secret cardiologist did not take the time to even determine who was actually being accused. In addition, he discounted the importance of Alex avoiding running. This is parallel to the comments made by the older cardiologist during the 3 days of my son's dying in Hospital 1 after his cardiac arrest. *The older cardiologist stated to me that running was not a factor in my son's death. You may recall that this limitation was left out of the letter from the electrophysiologist to the older cardiologist (Exhibit 5B).* Allow me to do a little armchair probability calculation on the risk from running and SCD.

Assuming that my son ran about 1 hour each day and knowing that his syncope occurred while he was running, the chances that his syncope randomly occurred while he was running was about 1/24 on any given day. Furthermore, if he ran an hour on the day he died and he died while running, then the chance that his cardiac arrest was unrelated to running (random) was 1/24. If I further assume the obvious, that his syncope and SCD were related, then the chance that running was unrelated to either of these events (syncope and sudden death) is less than 1 in 500 (1/[24×24]). So, one can conclude that anyone, cardiologists included, who claims that running and my son's death were unrelated has about a 1 in 500 chance of being right and about a 499 in 500 chance of being wrong. *A ban on running mattered, it mattered that Alex be told this in writing, it mattered that he be told at his follow-up visit (with the PIT) not to run, and to deny that these things mattered is unconscionable.* It also mattered if Alex had the genetic form of LQTS as the electrophysiologist had speculated after his EP testing. A cardiology textbook states, "Competitive sports are contraindicated for patients with the congenital LQTS" (Olgin and Zipes, 2001). In my final letter to the director of the TMB, in May of 2005, I concluded that *"by stating that my son's medical care exceeded the standard for medical care, he [the 2nd secret cardiologist] made a mockery of your process and his profession."*

A Friend's Story

In the summer of 2005, my surviving son and I were planning to go on a bus trip into the mountains of Colorado with one of the ministers of our church. The church group consisted primarily of two dozen teenagers with a few adults sprinkled in for control. We were loading the bus on Sunday after church when one of the older boys said that he might not be able to make the trip because his dad might have some heart problems. I knew this young man fairly well because he had been in a bible study I had been teaching at my house, and I also knew his older sister from mission trips. This was a family that was very easy to like. I found his mom and asked what the health situation was with her husband. She said it was thought that her husband had a heart condition and that tomorrow (Monday) he was to have a catheterization or EP test. I asked if she had gotten a second opinion about the need for this test, and she said no. I told her that the risk of serious complications from these tests was not trivial, and that the risk of death, from my reading, was one in several hundred. I urged her to get a second opinion before the testing began. In the meantime, she had decided that her son should go on the Colorado adventure, and so he did. Here is my friend's story in his own words:

"On Wednesday afternoon I began to have slight discomfort in the center of my abdomen. When I went home after work the discomfort had grown. After several hours I ended up in bed with severe pain. My wife drove me to the local hospital, where they looked at my pain location, age, and weight, and started to treat me for the possibility of a heart attack.

My past medical history is that I had had PVCs for several years before this event and I see a cardiologist. I take lisinopril (an ACE inhibitor) to make my heart work more efficiently and Lipitor for high cholesterol. Previous ECGs continued to show the PVCs. I have had several stress tests with normal results and echocardiography studies showing no significant problems.

In the emergency room I was given aspirin as a precaution for a heart attack and morphine for the pain. A short time later I was laid flat and given nitroglycerin under my tongue. About this time a technician came in to take an X-ray. He sat me up to put the film behind my back. Just as he put the film behind my back, the nitroglycerin under my tongue seemed to "burst" under my tongue. I recall telling the technician I was going to faint, which I then did. My wife was present just outside the emergency room looking in through glass windows. The next thing I recall was the nurse telling me it was time to wake up. I was then admitted to an intensive care room for the next two days. I rested pretty comfortably the first night with only the slight discomfort in the center of my abdomen. They connected me to a remote monitor to track my ECG until I left the hospital.

The next morning my cardiologist arrived and told me the results of my first blood test. This blood test did not confirm a heart attack, but he said the first test sometimes was inconclusive. He ordered a second blood test and an echocardiography study. He also told me that during the fainting incident in the emergency room, my heart stopped for 8 seconds and he needed to find out what caused this heart stoppage.

The echo showed little change from my previous echoes. The second blood test also did not confirm a heart attack. My cardiologist then ordered a heart catheterization and started to discuss the need for an EP study of the heart. The hospital I was at was equipped to do the heart catheterization, but I would have to be transferred to another hospital for the EP study.

Late Thursday afternoon, the heart catheterization was done. The results showed no blockages. That evening I was in great pain while I had to lie flat on my back for a long period to control the bleeding from the wound where the catheter was inserted. The pain was again located in the center of my abdomen. After about 40 minutes I was able to slightly sit up and the pain subsided.

Friday, about noon, my cardiologist told me the third blood test results concluded I had not had a heart attack. He also told me that he would admit me to a regular room at the hospital for the weekend for observation and have me transferred to the other hospital for the EP study to be done by a specialist and, depending on the results, a pacemaker would be inserted. He was still concerned about the 8-second heart stoppage while I was in the emergency room. My cardiologist also told me he was leaving town that afternoon for the following week and his associate would follow up with me over the weekend. As he was leaving, I asked him if any of the treatment I had had could explain the discomfort I was still having in my abdomen. He then ordered an echo of this area for late Friday afternoon.

My son was scheduled to go on a church trip for the following week. My wife dropped him off. While she was there a friend heard of my problems and relayed his past experience with doctors and his son's death. He advised us to continue to question the doctors, get a second opinion, and make sure we were comfortable with the recommended treatment. He explained the EP heart study procedure and how serious it was.

Saturday afternoon my cardiologist's associate arrived to check in on me. He told me that my EP heart study was scheduled for Monday morning. As he was leaving, I asked him about the results of the echo that was done late Friday afternoon on my abdomen. He did not know about this test and went to the nurse's station for the results. He came back a short time later and told me I had gallstones. He then arranged for the staff surgeon to talk to me about gallbladder surgery. The surgeon said my gallbladder was severely inflamed with multiple gallstones. He believed that the gallbladder was the source of the initial pain that brought me to the emergency room.

My wife and I began to question the need for the EP heart study. We talked by phone to the doctor who was scheduled to do the test. He continued to insist the study was needed due to the 8-second heart stoppage. My wife then tried to get an informal second opinion from a cardiologist who was the father of one of my son's friends. Late Sunday evening, this doctor returned to town. He thought we should take the time to get a formal second opinion.

My wife and I did not know how to proceed late Sunday night. We decided to go ahead and transfer to the other hospital in preparation for the surgery, but before the surgery we would again talk with the specialist about the need for the EP test.

When they transferred me to the other hospital, they also sent my medical file. My wife knew now that we had the right to review that file. Since we had nothing to do but wait, we asked to see it. The file had two glaring errors in it. The first one was that I had to be resuscitated in the emergency room when I fainted. The impression we got from this file was that they had to shock my heart to restart it. My wife said the only thing they did was pat my head. The other error was the report of a previous heart catheterization that had very poor results. I had never had a previous heart catheterization.

With this information, we insisted on talking to the doctor scheduled to perform the EP study of the heart. He told us (via the nurse) that he had already talked to us and that if we did not want the scheduled test, he was not going to come in. We then decided to cancel the test and get a second opinion. Shortly after this, his assistant and later a nurse asked us why we canceled my **pacemaker** surgery. We checked out of the hospital about noon.

A couple of days later we gathered all the files, test results, and films and gave them to another doctor for a second opinion. We met him later that week. He had talked to several other doctors about my history. All of them agreed that the EP study was not justified and that the 8-second stoppage was most likely due to a combination of the morphine, nitroglycerin, and being sat up at the wrong time.

This doctor cleared me for abdominal surgery and I had my gallbladder removed the following week. It has now been about 10 months since my gallbladder surgery and I have not had any other medical problems since. I have also changed cardiologists to the doctor who gave me the second opinion."

Austen's Story

In the final days of 2006, my wife persuaded me to have our younger son evaluated for the possibility of a genetic form of LQTS. He had chosen to play a physically demanding sport (lacrosse), and so there was some concern that the older cardiologist's belated assertion that Alex did not have a genetic disease could be in error. Although I was confident that this was one of the few things the older cardiologist had gotten right, I agreed, and we obtained an appointment with a pediatric cardiologist who served our area of Houston. We were asked to bring in Alex's pathology report. We brought that in along with his ECGs from August 19 and August 20. During our office visit I made it clear that I had studied Alex's medical records and the medical literature, and I had a strongly-held opinion of what caused his death. I did not say what my opinion was. The cardiologist looked at the pathology report for about a minute and then at the 2 ECGs for another minute and declared: It looks to me like Alex probably had LQTS. I said that I agreed with him, and that in my opinion he had the acquired form due to hypokalemia. The pediatric cardiologist said that there are forms of LQTS that do not show complete genetic penetrance, thus there is only a susceptibility to the disease. I said that if he saw Alex's other ECGs, including one from the Air Force, and his potassium levels, he would understand why I was confident that Alex had the acquired form of LQTS.

Why was this cardiologist prepared to diagnose LQTS when all the cardiologists called upon to review Alex's records were evasive about this diagnosis? I believe the answer is that the context of the pediatric cardiologist's evaluation was not threatening to another cardiologist, whereas the contexts of all the other evaluations were threatening to their colleagues. This observation led me to a remarkable insight into how to deal with physician bias when one of their own is accused. I'll share that with you in Chapter 10.

The pediatric cardiologist made an interesting, unsolicited comment about the Dallas pathologist, whom he knew. He said he knew the man to be "bombastic." This is an unusual word that I seldom hear. The last time I heard it was as a characterization of Saddam Hussein's behavior during his murder trial in Iraq. It is easy to forget that members of the physician community know each other surprisingly well.

Chapter 4
The Dallas Pathologist: A Doctor's Doctor?

The Pathology—Making a Scapegoat

In ancient biblical times a scapegoat was the second of 2 goats brought to the sacrificial altar once each year for the atonement of sins committed by the people. The first goat was offered as a blood sacrifice, but the priest placed his hands on the second one and symbolically imparted all the people's sins to the goat. That goat was then freed to run off, carrying all the sins of the people away. And so it was that the Dallas pathologist selected by the older cardiologist to examine Alex's heart was able to find a scapegoat to carry away the sins of the people, in this case Alex's doctors. I should point out that if my son had gone into a sustained coma as Terri Schiavo did, then his heart would not have been available immediately for examination by a pathologist, and I believe his cardiologists probably would have been held accountable for their many mistakes. But evidence of disease (pathology) was found in his heart...

The pathologist's report came 3 months after my son died (December 2002) and was received by my first lawyer, who called me with the news. When I saw the report I was livid for 2 reasons. The lie about Alex and his parents refusing a pacemaker had been spread even into this pathologist's report, and the report was obviously based on a hurried, superficial effort. The pathologist noted abnormal changes in structure (lesions) in the subendocardial septum, in the papillary muscles, and in the subepicardial layer of the left ventricle, but he took thin sections to examine with a microscope from only the subepicardial lesions (Exhibit 10). These he characterized from gross observation (without a microscope) as "consistent with...healing myocarditis." The words "consistent with" are weasel words sometimes used by doctors or scientists when they are not certain of what the entity in question actually is. The gross lesions, and also the description of their microscopic structure, were consistent with other disease processes besides myocarditis. I will show you that momentarily.

Myocarditis is an inflammation of the heart muscle. The most common cause is believed to be viral infection; however, other causes are known. It may be first detected as an abnormality in the ECG, or the patient may have vague chest pain and shortness of breath. Most people recover completely from the acute illness, especially if the heart is rested; however, in some cases it may progress to a more serious disease when scar tissue is deposited in the heart or the heart muscle dilates. The histological definition of myocarditis may vary, but it is reasonably commonly found at routine autopsy of hospitalized patients (Gravanis and Sternby, 1991).

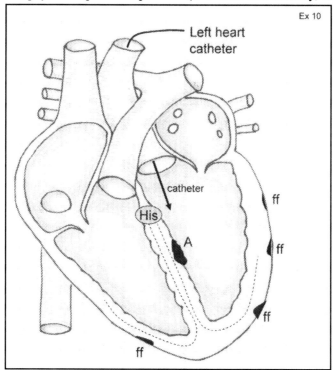

Exhibit 10. Approximate locations of heart lesions found by the Dallas pathologist. The acute subendocardial lesion is marked "A" and the subepicardial focal fibrosis is marked "ff."

Microscopic sections will show the formation of scar tissue and bead-like cells near areas of dying (necrotic) tissue. Diagnosis of this condition requires the demonstration of 20 to 30 inflammatory cells per high-power field in the microscope around areas of necrotic tissue (Phillips et al., 1986). During the months after I received his report, I had repeatedly asked this pathologist to show or state to me that the lesion he looked at fit this standard definition of myocarditis and he steadfastly refused. After I had made repeated attempts to extract details from this man, he admitted to me in a phone conversation on January 11, 2006, that the lesions in Alex's heart did not meet the standard definition above; that's why he called it "healing" myocarditis.

The pathologist's report had many other shortcomings besides his ill-defined "myocarditis" and his insertion of the statement about the pacemaker, which I proved to him was false. I asked him to remove the pacemaker statement from his report after sending him copies of Alex's medical records from Hospital 2, which clearly showed that a loop monitor was offered and not a pacemaker, but he refused to correct his records, deciding instead to keep my letter in his files. *To me his attitude reflected the irrelevance of truth among physicians when one of their own is accused. It made me think that protecting the community of physicians is most important to physicians even when truth must suffer.*

Perhaps the pathologist's most glaring mistake is that he did not examine microscopic sections of the other gross lesions he had observed, in the left ventricle's subendocardial septum and in the papillary muscles. Microscopic observation of such lesions is essential to determine their age by the amount of scar tissue and their possible role in causing death by their proximity to critical structures in the heart. In my profession of toxicology, when we expose animals to a potentially toxic material, federal government regulations called "good laboratory practices" require the study pathologist (usually a veterinary pathologist) to make a microscope slide of *any* lesion that is grossly observed during necropsy (animal autopsy) of the exposed animal, typically a rat or mouse (EPA, 2001). I have asked my human pathologist colleagues at the agency where I work if they are aware of standards for making a decision on when to make a microscope slide during a human autopsy and when not to. They are not aware of any standards for this. *Thus, pathologically speaking, there is more regulatory control and deeper evaluation of dead rats than dead children.*

I have asked the Dallas pathologist a number of questions over the years since his initial report was released, some of which he has been gracious enough to answer. In one of his answers he stated, "I think a viral etiology is speculation." Another of his answers had to do with the age of the lesions he characterized as healing "myocarditis." He stated, "I would tend to estimate the myocardial lesions to be well over 2 months old." This is consistent with the words I finally extracted from him that the lesions did not fit the standard definition for myocarditis. He has refused to answer the following important questions:

1) Given the healed or healing nature of the lesions, would you have expected them to worsen over time?
2) Could the subepicardial lesions be better characterized as "idiopathic (cause unknown) myocardial scarring?" This is a cardiac lesion described in an article called "Sudden death in young competitive athletes" in *JAMA* (Maron et al., 1996). That article states, "Four of the athletes showed only isolated areas of idiopathic myocardial scarring, which could conceivably represent the healing phase of myocarditis."

3) In an earlier letter you stated that the subepicardial lesions precipitated Alex's death. Since his syncope and SCD occurred while he was running, wouldn't it be more accurate to state that running precipitated his death?

4) Can you offer any pathological explanation for the disappearance of the 3 risk factors for SCD from my son's ECG in an 8-hour period [August 19-20]?

5) He stated in a letter to me, "I believe that they [the acute lesions] occurred after the cardiac arrest and that they played no part in the cardiac arrest." Since there were acute lesions in 2 locations, I asked during my final phone discussion with him if the most likely cause of the acute lesions inside the left ventricular septum was trauma from left heart catheterization. The pathologist did tell me that the lesions in the papillary muscles were probably from oxygen deprivation, but he refused to comment on the cause of the lesions in Alex's left ventricular septum.

Answers to all these questions are crucial because they go to the question of whether the old lesions were progressive and would have eventually caused my son's death even if his potassium had been corrected, or could the lesions have been stabilized or even reversed? In the absence of any clear answers from the Dallas pathologist, I had some insight as a Ph.D. pathologist. Although conventional thinking is that scar tissue in the heart will remain regardless of therapy, this is not entirely supported by the medical literature. Since the 1940s, studies (such as Schrader et al., 1937 in Tepper et al., 1990; Mergner et al., 1984) have been published showing that hypomagnesemia and/or hypokalemia can cause cardiomyopathy (physical injury to the heart muscle), especially if catecholamines (a hormone produced during running or other vigorous activity) are elevated (Rowe, 1992). There is a peer-reviewed publication about animal studies called "Recovery of heart tissue following focal injury induced by dietary restriction of potassium" (Tepper et al., 1990). In this study rats were fed a potassium-deficient diet for 42 days and found to have *small areas (foci) of heart muscle cell necrosis infiltrated by mononuclear cells and having early evidence of fibrosis (an excess of collagen fibers and the fibroblasts that make them)*, but when the potassium was replaced for only 6 days, the lesions entirely disappeared except for a limited scar. I ask you to compare this description of hypokalemic cardiomyopathy with the Dallas pathologist's description of the lesion in my son's heart: "*focal replacement fibrosis and rare focus of mononuclear cells associated with*

myofiber necrosis. " The lesion found in my son's heart is fully consistent with hypokalemic cardiomyopathy!

Furthermore, even in cardiology textbooks, statements have been published such as "in patients with hypomagnesemia, focal myocardial necrosis may occur...ventricular arrhythmias often develop, including serious ventricular arrhythmias. Repletion of magnesium usually corrects these arrhythmias" (Willerson, 1995). Thus there is compelling evidence that if my son's cardiologists had recognized and treated his electrolyte problems according to the medical standard (Cohn et al., 2000), or provided therapy in response to a diagnosis of acquired LQTS (Khan, 2002), he would be alive and well today. This information allows the addition of new lines to the figure relating stress (running) to functional (electrolyte) and structural (fibrosis) cardiac illnesses. As Figure 7 shows, if the hypokalemia and hypomagnesemia are corrected, at least part of the stimulus to scarring is gone and the fibrosis could at least partially reverse.

You will notice that I have added "poor diet" to the diagram. This is application of Tool 6, by which you know that a diet poor in fruits and vegetables can lead to depletion of potassium and magnesium. A good-quality medical history on my son would have revealed that he seldom ate fruits or vegetables. A nutritional history is important when an electrolyte imbalance is suspected, and standard formats for this had been available in the medical literature for at least 3 years before his death (Hark and Deen, 1999). During the 4 days of his hospital evaluation, he would have had plenty of time to fill out a standard form. This would have shown his distaste for rich sources of potassium. I recall with some sadness that the last email I ever sent Alex gave a list of potassium-rich foods that I had gotten from a nutritionist colleague. About the only thing on the list that I thought he might eat was canned peaches. I was surprised to learn how many fruits and vegetables one must eat to ensure adequate potassium intake.

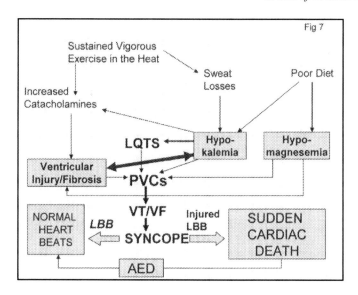

Figure 7. More complete model of sudden cardiac death showing that hypokalemia can cause fibrosis and how running, hypomagnesemia, and LQTS can play a role. Each relationship between the factors, shown by lines or arrows, has been demonstrated in peer-reviewed medical literature. The double-tipped arrow connecting fibrosis and hypokalemia indicates that fibrosis has the potential to be partially reversed if the hypokalemia is corrected. If the left bundle branch (LBB) is injured, then syncope is more likely to end in sudden death rather than a return to normal heart beats. Sometimes an AED can shock the heart back to "normal" heartbeats.

The realization that my son's myocardial lesions would have been at least partly reversible if electrolyte therapy had been administered was not a welcome discovery. I had supposed, before this discovery, that even if his electrolyte imbalance had been corrected and he took a break from running to rest his heart, he might have eventually begun to have more heart problems. Deep inside I still wanted to believe that his cardiologists' mistakes of omission had not resulted in his death, but that opinion was becoming impossible to maintain in the face of such evidence. More unsettling news was yet to come, but first the scapegoat needs to be hunted down.

Slaying the Scapegoat with Evidence-Based Medicine

The "myocarditis" scapegoat had been released and in the end did carry away the sins of the doctors because they were never held accountable for their many mistakes. The fundamental test question in such a case is that regardless of the number and severity of the errors made by the physicians, if they had gotten it right, would the patient have lived? Thus it was a convenient scapegoat for all physicians involved to simply state that my son's "myocarditis" killed him, and that no matter what tests were performed his doctors were unlikely to discover that disease. At face value it is true that myocarditis is a difficult diagnosis to make in life; however, a competent examination of the medical record will show that "myocarditis" simply set my son's heart up to be sensitive to hypokalemia and might have been at least partially reversed, as I showed above, if his electrolyte imbalances had been corrected.

The extent of scarring in Alex's heart suggests that the lesions there were relevant to his death, but they were not the controlling factor. The medical record proves, as much as anything can be proven in medicine, that untreated hypokalemia was the root cause of Alex's syncope. This can be deduced from the appearance and disappearance of risk factors present in his ECGs. *There is no way that any changes in his subepicardial heart lesions (called myocarditis) in an 8-hour period (2353 August 19 to 0736 August 20) could have eliminated his PVCs, corrected his LQTS, and normalized his QTd. The only explanation for this is the rise in his serum potassium from 3.4 to 3.9 mmol/L, which was simultaneous with the disappearance of these risk factors. This is equivalent to removing the right–hand portion of the stimulus to PVCs in Figure 7, and it explains why Alex did fine on his exercise stress test after his syncope. Furthermore, if he had stopped running, as the cardiologists told him while he was sedated but never wrote down for him, then the potassium losses and catecholamine stimulus would have ceased.* In the analysis below I will show this in some detail, and back it up with medical literature. But first I would like the reader to play investigator for a moment with the pathology data. Pretend you are "Quincy," or if you prefer, "Jordan." Many of the clues have already been given to deduce the ultimate cause of Alex's death; perhaps the careful reader has already pieced those clues together. Potassium mattered, a ban on running mattered, but something else more sinister was going on.

First Do No Harm: Was There a Killer?

A few weeks before the 3rd anniversary of Alex's death, I began to deal with one final question that had troubled me since his death: Why did he self-recover from his first collapse, maximize the exercise stress test 2 days later, and then only 3 weeks later die after he collapsed again while running? What had changed about his heart in those weeks that prevented it from self-recovery the second time he collapsed? Each time he was running or doing vigorous exercise, so that alone cannot explain the difference in outcome. The so-called "myocarditis" was healed or healing at the time of his death and was estimated to be "well over 2 months old" by the Dallas pathologist, so that lesion does not explain the difference. Then I recalled something my pathologist friend (this man is a world-class pathologist I know from working with him on the National Research Council of the National Academy of Sciences) had written to me in the spring of 2003 after examining microscope slides of Alex's heart and apparently discussing the case with the Dallas pathologist: "At the time of postmortem examination [of Alex's heart], there were acute lesions noted in the left ventricular papillary muscles and in the subendocardial region of the ventricular septum....It has been my experience that inflammatory processes which involve the subendocardial region of the ventricular septum, may disturb the electrophysiology of the ventricle since the Purkinje system is in this area." This is exactly the lesion that the Dallas pathologist had refused to examine under the microscope. *If the Purkinje system had been injured between his syncope and fatal collapse, then this would explain why Alex died the second time he collapsed and not the first. From Tool 1, you know how close these structures are.*

Once a PVC occurs, it is up to the normal electrical system of the heart to reestablish useful heartbeats. The normal system, which passes electrical impulses through the ventricular septum, must override the ventricle's tendency to beat on its own without accepting impulses from the normal electrical system. If the ability of the normal system to do this has been reduced (say by injury), then the ventricle will continue to produce PVCs until ventricular tachycardia, ventricular fibrillation, and sudden cardiac death ensue (Figure 7). This is consistent with my colleague's opinion as a pathologist.

I will now provide you with facts from my son's medical records and from medical literature and ask that you deduce the cause of this potentially fatal lesion in the subendocardial region of the left ventricular septum. This time you, dear reader, are the pathologist in search of a killer. Here are your clues:

1) The complications from left heart catheterization, as listed on the consent form my son signed, include the following: bleeding at the site of vessel puncture (hematoma), heart attack, and sudden death. The hospital website adds other complications to include heart perforation. The case report by Marine et al. (2001) describes a catheter-induced lesion precisely on the interventricular septum, and this caused persistent His-Purkinje system injury, just as my pathologist friend had noted in his letter to me.

2) During Alex's left heart catheterization, the older cardiologist used a 7F catheter, which is much larger in diameter and stiffer than the normally used 4F or 5F catheters (Mitty, 2003; Kern et al., 1990). In 1999, 4F and 5F catheter use became the norm and continues today (Lim, 2005).

3) Larger-diameter catheters are known to cause a higher risk of trauma and hematoma than their smaller counterparts (Harrison, 2001; Lee et al., 2000; Lim, 2005).

4) A few hours after his catheterization, the medical record shows that Alex had a hematoma, which is an unusual complication.

5) Alex's resting ECGs done on the 20th and 21st showed no PVCs. During his exercise stress test the day *before the catheterization*, the cardiologist noted an *occasional* PVC, which is not unusual during exercise.

6) Of the 18 limited ECGs analyzed by the nursing staff of Hospital 1 between 1300 on August 20 and Alex's discharge late in the evening of August 22, only 1 showed any PVCs (Exhibit 8, page 41), and this was the only routine monitoring to show PVCs with different-shaped PVCs (multiform). This record was made a few hours *after* his catheterization. Nothing in the medical record of the catheterization procedure suggests that an injury took place. Sporadic records of other PVCs are noted in his records, and 3 other nursing staff ECGs taken after his catheterization did not show PVCs.

7) One day *after the catheterization*, the electrophysiologist doing the EP testing noted in his medical record that Alex now had *frequent* ventricular ectopy (PVCs).

8) The only foreign objects that entered Alex's left ventricle in his entire life were the catheter, wire, and dye used during his left heart catheterization.

9) Alex's ventricular septum was thin, according to the results of the echocardiogram done on August 20 (0.73 cm, outside the adult normal range of 0.8 to 1.1 cm) (see Exhibit 7, page 41).

10) Subendocardial lesions were not noted on the right side of Alex's ventricular septum, suggesting that any general trauma to his heart, which would have affected both sides, was not the cause of the lesion on the left side of the septum. Rupture (making a hole from the left to the right side) of the ventricular septum is a rare complication reported after myocardial infarction (Antmann and Braunwald, 2001).

11) The maximum effects of a heart tissue injury may not be manifested until several weeks *after* the injury occurred because scar tissue increases over a period of several weeks, and *then* affects nearby structures such as the His-Purkinje system. Alex's catheterization was done on August 22 and his fatal collapse occurred on September 15.

12) The older cardiologist was busy, performing catheterizations at a rate of 450 per year (personal communication to me from the catheterization lab).

The following is not a fact; however, it provides perspective to you. I work with a veterinarian whose mother needed to have a left heart catheterization some time after Alex died. This veterinarian was well connected to physicians working at the medical centers in Houston. Before allowing her mother to undergo this procedure, she searched for a cardiologist with a reputation for doing gentle as opposed to "brutish" cardiac catheterizations. She found such a cardiologist and as far as I know her mother's cardiac catheterization took place with no evident trauma. My point is that there are large variations in the approach cardiologists take when performing cardiac catheterizations.

Is this factual and perspective-type evidence sufficient to identify the probable ultimate cause of death? I think it is. Of course if you or I were "Quincy" or "Jordan," we would have taken a section of the lesion in question and examined it under the microscope. The Dallas pathologist could not be bothered.

Chapter 5
Evaluation by an Informed Cardiologist

The reader has been subjected to a troubling and at times difficult journey through cardiology and my son's treatment. In this section I will indicate, by summarizing and introducing a few new medical references, how I think an informed, unbiased, careful cardiologist or pathologist would have evaluated the medical care my son received at the hands of his physicians. I will use only information provided to the 5 cardiologists (counting the chairman of the DPRC) involved in evaluating Alex's medical records. *I want you to understand that the combination of being uninformed in cardiology and being unwilling to criticize an uninformed colleague is a deadly combination that leaves patients incredibly vulnerable to ongoing mistakes by physicians.* The time for physicians to be in control of who is held accountable for medical mistakes must end. Here is truth as I see it.

Alex was the victim of uninformed, inattentive, inexperienced, and unethical medical care by a loose group of physicians who failed to communicate clearly with each other and with their young patient. The weight of evidence is that his life would have been saved if his cardiologists had recognized his overt hypokalemia (3.4 mmol/L) and borderline low magnesium as the cause of 2 manageable risk factors he had for sudden cardiac death (SCD). Those risk factors were present in his ECG taken immediately after he collapsed while running on August 19. The first factor was the presence of PVCs in his resting ECG soon after his syncope, and the second was the presence of a prolonged QTc interval (479 ms). Although most PVCs are benign, they are known to be the gateway to SCD (Myerburg and Castellanos, 2001), and prolonged QT intervals are associated with a higher risk of SCD (Choy et al., 1997). Both are known to be sensitive to hypokalemia (Moss, 1993; Castellanos et al., 2001).

The consulting cardiologist from Austin noted these 2 risk factors in the record; however, he did not note their disappearance in the ECG taken only 8 hours later when Alex's potassium had been normalized (3.9 mmol/L). This failure to compare the ECGs was a catastrophic oversight. Unfortunately, the record shows that the consulting cardiologist took Alex's initial QTc to be upper normal at 490 ms, which is another catastrophic error. Any informed cardiologist should know that a QTc above 450 ms is abnormal in a young man. Chou and Knilans (1996) state, "In patients without evidence of cardiac dysfunction, a QTc interval of more than 440 ms was associated with a 2-3 times higher risk for sudden death compared with those patients with a QTc interval of 440 ms or less." In an article in *The Physician and Sports Medicine* (Vincent, 1998), the author observes, "The average QTc interval for someone who has LQTS is 490 ms, an abnormal value that is generally not obvious on casual observation of an ECG."

A third risk factor that disappeared was Alex's high dispersion in QT intervals. His QTd dropped from 120 ms in his August 19 ECG to only 40 ms in his ECG taken 8 hours later on August 20. A QTd of 120 ms is an extremely abnormal value, far exceeding any published normal upper limits, which are consistently below 70 ms (Mirvis and Goldberger, 2001; Perkiomaki et al., 1997; Castellanos et al., 2001). Many articles citing the association between QTd and SCD in infarct patients were published in the mid-1990s. Four of these were cited in an article entitled "Sudden death due to cardiac arrhythmias" published in the *New England Journal of Medicine* (Huikuri et al., 2001). The dispersion of QT values in an ECG is easily calculated if the cardiologists simply take the time to do the measurements.

All 3 of these risk factors are associated with hypokalemia and/or hypomagnesemia and all 3 disappeared when Alex's potassium was elevated by 0.5 mmol/L into the low normal range. It has been shown that the magnitude of decrease in Alex's QT interval (90 ms) can be directly caused by an increase in the blood potassium of about half a mmol/L in cardiology patients (Choy et al., 1997). *The failure of Alex's doctors to recognize the presence of 3 risk factors for SCD and an obvious way to manage them is practicing dangerously uninformed and inattentive cardiology.*

Noting that Alex had a normal QTc in his March 2002 ECG and again after his hypokalemia normalized on August 20, and applying the Schwartz criteria for diagnosis of LQTS to the August 19 ECG, or simply knowing that a normal QTc interval is less than 450 ms, confirms the diagnosis of acquired LQTS (Schwartz et al., 1993). In reference to the diagnosis of LQTS, Schwartz et al. (2000) make the following statement in a cardiology textbook: *"The unusual combination of an often lethal disease for which effective therapies exist and of a rather elementary diagnosis makes inexcusable the existence of undiagnosed, and therefore untreated, patients [with LQTS]."* The fact that Alex was a runner and in the military brings to bear the report that under such conditions (vigorous exercise in hot conditions) potassium depletion is a real possibility (Knochel et al., 1972). I would not have expected his cardiologists to know this specific cause; however, it provides an explanation for his potassium depletion and associated diagnosis of *acquired* LQTS.

The association of a prolonged QTc and sudden death has been known for decades (Isner et al., 1979). A cardiology textbook published 5 years before Alex's death summarizes the importance of diagnosing and treating acquired LQTS very well (Myerburg and Castellanos, 1997): *"Acquired prolonged Q-T intervals usually carry a risk of serious arrhythmias and SCD, but the risk is abolished when the inciting factor is removed. In acquired prolonged Q-T syndrome, as in the congenital form, the torsades de pointes form of ventricular tachycardia is commonly the specific arrhythmia that triggers or degenerates into lethal ventricular fibrillation."* Torsades de points literally means a twisting of the heart muscle.

Alex's physicians not only failed to recognize his initial hypokalemia, they were remiss in not ordering a magnesium determination, and then when they finally did that after his stress test and found it to be borderline low, they failed to ask for a magnesium determination from the laboratory where the post-syncope blood sample was stored. The relationship between hypokalemia and hypomagnesemia is extremely well known, and magnesium depletion, which can occur in the presence of low normal serum magnesium, has been thoroughly associated with heart disease for decades (Seelig, 1980). Restoration of magnesium is often necessary to fully correct potassium depletion (Sica et al., 2002). Furthermore, a wise cardiologist would have ordered a panel of cardiac enzymes to detect any ongoing cell injury or death (Antman and Braunwald, 2001). Alex's ECGs did clearly suggest the possibility of cardiac tissue injury.

Failure to note the disappearance of these risk factors from Alex's ECG, and failure to diagnose acquired LQTS due to hypokalemia (and possibly hypomagnesemia) were catastrophic mistakes, but not ones that could not have been overcome if his cardiologists had been informed and attentive to a clinical practice guideline for potassium replacement published in 2000. That guideline mandates potassium replacement and monitoring in patients with arrhythmias and potassium levels below 4.0 mmol/L (Cohn et al., 2000). Alex had PVCs and a long QT interval (506 ms), which are arrhythmias, and his potassium was only 3.4 mmol/L. *Even without the obvious proper diagnosis of acquired LQTS, if his cardiologists had followed the guideline for arrhythmia and potassium replacement, his life would have been saved.* Not long before Alex had his cardiac evaluation, another group of physicians, "realizing the substantial risks of hypokalemia," suggested that patients with cardiac arrhythmias and normal renal function should maintain potassium levels from 4.5 to 5.0 mmol/L (Sica et al., 2002).

Failure to apply the guideline or diagnose acquired LQTS not only led Alex's physicians away from his correct diagnosis and treatment, it led them into unnecessary and painful invasive testing. However, *the record clearly shows that a cardiac MRI was to have been done before any invasive testing was undertaken, and that this is what Alex and his parents agreed to. Unfortunately, his medical record has nothing about the findings of any cardiac MRI, thus one must suspect that something was amiss with the result.* Furthermore, there is no evidence that any findings from the putative cardiac MRI were communicated to the patient. I note here that routine cardiac MRIs were being performed, often using gadolinium enhancer, at a nearby medical center in Dallas. If Hospital 1 was incapable of performing a clinically relevant cardiac MRI, then Alex should have been given the choice of going to Dallas. Guidelines for informed consent clearly require that the patient be informed of any reasonable choices he has to the proposed invasive testing (Bashore et al., 2001; AMA, 1998). No evidence exists in the record that this option was presented to him. *This withholding of critical information about the cardiac MRI from the patient suggests an unethical practice of medicine.*

The record shows that Alex's invasive left heart catheterization was performed by a cardiologist using unusually large 7F catheters, known to be more likely to cause trauma than the smaller and more commonly used 4F and 5F catheters that were the norm by the late 1990s (Harrison, 2001; Lim, 2005). Anyone who realized that the patient's potassium level had been temporarily corrected, probably by diurnal variation, and that all 3 risk factors for SCD had disappeared from his ECG would not have been surprised that the result was negative. The record also shows that Alex had a hematoma on his groin after this procedure. The risk of this is less than 1% when the procedure is carefully performed, thus suggesting that the cardiologist may have been careless in performing the catheterization. Of course, *since Alex's cardiologists had not deduced the proper diagnosis or treatment, the negative result of the catheterization was taken as a definitive finding rather than a transient finding, applicable only as long as his potassium was normalized.* It should be noted that the transient nature of Alex's underlying condition is apparent from his ability after his syncope, when his potassium had normalized, to perform the entire Bruce exercise protocol.

The second unnecessary invasive testing suffered by Alex was the electrophysiology test performed at Hospital 2. Clinical Practice Guidelines for EP testing state that EP testing is not justified in a class III situation (Zipes et al., 1995). These guidelines explicitly state in the "Class

III" column that EP testing is inappropriate in "patients with acquired prolonged QT syndrome and symptoms closely related to an identifiable cause or mechanism." Had Alex's acquired LQTS due to hypokalemia been properly diagnosed from the beginning, the EP testing would have been unjustified. This is why it was critical for the consulting cardiologist to know that a 490 ms QTc was abnormal, not upper normal as he stated in Alex's medical record. Although the EP test failed to induce any ventricular tachycardia, it did show "frequent ectopic activity," suggesting that Alex's prevalence of PVCs had increased compared to the prevalence established before the catheterization. It also showed an appropriate decrease in the QT interval with increasing heart rate, which argues against any diagnosis of genetic LQTS. Finally, Alex's doctors depended far too much on the results of the EP testing without careful and informed inspection of his ECGs from Hospital 1. *The transient hypokalemia that caused his syncope had been temporarily rectified, and EP testing can certainly give false negative results in such a situation* (Krahn et al., 1995).

The records from Hospital 2, where the EP testing was performed, show that Alex was told 3 things: have a loop monitor inserted, avoid vigorous activity for now, and have a genetic test for LQTS done by a doctor in Houston; however, the only information given to him in writing was to avoid driving for 24 hours. This proved to be a catastrophic oversight. *Failure to provide Alex with a written record of the recommendations told to him is a clear violation of medical standards for communication with a patient*. A letter from the electrophysiologist to the older cardiologist reiterates Alex's need for a loop monitor and genetic testing, but there is a strange absence of any words about avoiding vigorous activity. It is not clear what, if anything, more than oversight by the electrophysiologist prompted this deletion, but *it was a catastrophic error to allow Alex to return to running without any lasting treatment of his hypokalemia.* If the electrophysiologist had been right about the genetic cause of Alex's LQTS, then it was important for him to restrict vigorous activity until further resolution had been achieved (Vincent et al., 1998). Since Alex died while running, his physician's carelessness in this regard clearly contributed to his death.

The medical records attributed to the physician in training (hospital discharge and last office visit) suggest a careless attitude toward accuracy and possibly the fabrication of false statements. Her records are full of wrong statements and are missing crucial information, especially the change in Alex's ECGs. These summary medical records suggest that Alex and his parents refused an electroencephalogram, yet the only entry in the progress notes is that Alex's family asked if he needed a neurological evaluation and electroencephalogram. *It stretches the limits of credibility to suppose that Alex and his parents refused a non-invasive electroencephalogram and accepted the invasive catheterization and EP testing, which each have some risk of death.* The records from Hospital 2 and a letter from the electrophysiologist to the older cardiologist show that Alex was offered a loop monitor. *The suggestion that he was offered a pacemaker seems to me to be a fabrication, unless we are to believe that Alex was offered both of these devices and only the loop monitor was written in the medical record.* Evidence that the false statement about the pacemaker was deliberately spread to other physicians' records, and that they placed it in their records without verifying it, suggests a concerted effort to mislead any later attempt to evaluate the medical records and reach a truthful conclusion. It is a direct violation of the second point of the Hippocratic Oath adopted in 2001 by the AMA to lie to your physician colleagues in professional interactions.

Finally, the Dallas pathologist's report on Alex's heart and follow-up answers provided to Alex's father in a letter from the pathologist suggest that his study of the heart was uninformed, hurried, and incomplete, and that he exaggerated the value of his conclusions. It was uninformed in part because he did not have access to Alex's medical records. *If the cardiologists had been practicing pre-1975 cardiology (when LQTS was not yet recognized as a disease entity), then the pathologist was practicing pre-1700 pathology, before Anton van Leeuwenhoek learned to make incredibly good lenses and used them to discover the remarkable world of cells. There is no defense for the pathologist's failure to examine by microscopy the lesions he saw grossly on the papillary muscles and subendocardial left ventricular septum.* His report omits any mention that the patient had had a left heart catheterization, a possible cause of the septal lesions. His conclusion that the subepicardial lesions, which he did examine microscopically, precipitated Alex's death is a thoughtless exaggeration of what a pathologist can deduce without looking at the patient's medical records.

Myocardial scarring, which the pathologist called healing myocarditis, is a common finding in people who die of non-cardiac causes. Thus, the more likely precipitating event of Alex's death was running (a known heart stressor) against a background of untreated hypokalemia and injury to his ventricular septum, possibly from the unnecessary left heart catheterization. Furthermore, in *non-exercising* dogs, experimental hypokalemia causes myocardial tissue injury (elevated cardiac enzymes) when potassium levels drop below about 3.3 mmol/L, and the injury worsens with decreasing potassium (Sugiyama et al., 1988). The pathologist's conclusion is also inconsistent with the disappearance of 3 risk factors for SCD between the ECGs of August 19 and August 20, which he was obviously not aware of. Pathological changes cannot explain the disappearance of these risk factors; only the disappearance of hypokalemia can do that.

Animal studies suggest that hypokalemic cardiomyopathy, which the pathologist mistakenly called healing myocarditis, may well have been partially reversed by potassium replacement therapy (Tepper et al., 1990). The root cause of Alex's ventricular scarring was not infection. There is no evidence in Alex's medical records that he had an infection in August, and he had no clinical symptoms associated with myocarditis. In contrast, there is compelling evidence that he was hypokalemic. This, coupled with possible magnesium depletion and vigorous exercise, had caused slow accumulation of scar tissue on his ventricles. The proper name for the lesion found on the outside surfaces of Alex's left ventricle was hypokalemic cardiomyopathy.

The pathologist's additional comment that "A pacemaker was recommended to the patient at the time [of his syncope], but both the patient and his parents refused to have it inserted" does not belong in an unbiased pathologist's report even if it were true. This information has absolutely nothing to do with pathology and could not have been confirmed by him as a true statement. Indeed, the medical record clearly shows that the recommendation was for a loop monitor, not a pacemaker. Its presence in the report suggests that the pathologist was complicit toward absolving the cardiologists of any mistakes even if it meant placing unconfirmed information in his report. Unfortunately, the pathologist's physician-protective bias is further magnified by his failure to perform a microscopic examination of the subendocardial lesions in the left ventricular septum, which may have been iatrogenic (caused by physicians). There is no defense for this sort of careless pathology, especially in the case of the death of a young man.

The general quality of Alex's medical treatment and the records associated with that treatment is very simply reflected in the quality of Hospital 1's pathologist's report. I offer a part of that record without comment (Exhibit 11). I will let you see with your own eyes!

FINAL AUTOPSY DIAGNOSES
AUTOPSY NUMBER: A02-11
PATIENT'S NAME: JAMES, ALEX
AGE: 19 SEX: MALE RACE: CAUCASIAN
PHYSICIANS: <DELETED>
MEDICAL RECORD NUMBER: 000536411
DATE ADMITTED: 9/15/02
DATE EXPIRED: 9/18/02 at 2225
DATE OF AUTOPSY: 9/18/02 at approximately 0930

Exhibit 11. Autopsy report from Hospital 1.

In summary, Alex's cardiologists missed his obvious diagnosis of acquired LQTS, missed his need for potassium replacement according to a widely published medical guideline, failed to give him authentic informed consent for invasive testing, delegated his hospital discharge report and follow-up to an inexperienced physician in training, failed to provide critical written instructions to him after his EP testing, and probably contributed to his death by performing an unnecessary and injurious left heart catheterization. False information about his being offered an electroencephalogram and pacemaker was entered into his medical records by some of his doctors. The scarring found in his heart does explain why his heart was sensitive to hypokalemia; indeed, the scarring was likely the result of hypokalemia (also hypomagnesemia) and vigorous exercise over many months. The pathologist should have called it hypokalemic cardiomyopathy, but he did not have access to Alex's medical records to know he was hypokalemic. Alex was the victim of grossly uninformed and unethical medical practice, and his death could have easily been prevented.

Chapter 6
Government Secrets

You might suppose that government entities exist to help protect patients from uninformed and unethical physicians. You would be wrong.

The Texas Medical Board (TMB) Process

Since I began interacting with this group in February 2004, it has changed its name from the Texas State Board of Medical Examiners to the Texas Medical Board (TMB). Its stated goal has not changed, however. That stated goal is as follows:

Our mission is to protect and enhance the public's health, safety and welfare by establishing and maintaining standards of excellence used in regulating the practice of medicine and ensuring quality health care for the citizens of Texas through licensure, discipline, and education.

The TMB is called upon to investigate patient complaints against physicians, and then a subgroup of the TMB, the DPRC, determines if the complaint has merit. There is often a strong imbalance between the knowledge, statements, and presentation skills of the complainants and any physicians involved. The situation is often extremely emotional for the patient or family of the victim and it is often adversarial in nature. If you were selecting persons to participate in the process of deciding if a physician harmed a patient, whom would you place on the medical board to ensure that the stated goal of protecting the patient is achieved? In other words, ***is there a presence on the DPRC that could act as a strong advocate for complainants, or is the deck stacked against the complaining patient or family member?*** I ask you to decide.

At the time my interaction with the TMB began, this group was composed of the following persons: 12 physicians (9 M.D.s and 3 D.O.s), and 7 non-physician public members: an administrative assistant, a public relations consultant, a director of community projects, a social research advisor, a recruiter and business developer, a realtor, and a business development consultant. Eight of the 12 physicians were men and 2 of the 7 non-physicians were men. I would argue that the deck was heavily stacked against any complainant for the following three reasons:

1) There are many more physicians than non-physicians on the board.

2) The proportion of men, who tend to be more assertive than women on average, among the physicians (67%) was much higher than among the non-physicians (30%). I note this with apologies to all women, especially some I know who are quite assertive.

3) None of the 7 non-physicians was technically oriented.

Does this situation result in a bias against the complainant and for any physician accused of wrongdoing?

Although I was warned by a physician friend that I was unlikely to receive justice from the TMB, I had no idea how much the deck was stacked against me as I began to pursue a complaint against the older cardiologist, the consulting cardiologist, and the PIT. I alleged that the older cardiologist disregarded medical standards for diagnosis and treatment, failed to obtain informed consent by not telling my son about the aborted MRI, and attempted to falsify the medical records by misleading his colleagues about a pacemaker being offered to Alex. I alleged that the consulting cardiologist's failure to make a proper diagnosis of acquired LQTS contributed to failure to give Alex the treatment he needed, and I alleged that the PIT had falsified her records of his office visit. Only my allegations of failure to follow medical standards and failure to make a life-saving diagnosis require technical expertise; however, it seems that if an allegation is against a cardiologist, then a secret cardiologist is in the critical path toward justice. This secret individual reviews the medical records of the alleged victim and renders a secret opinion as to whether medical standards have been followed. It is unclear to me whether any investigation ever occurred regarding my allegation of no informed consent or falsification of the medical records. ***This brings me to a 4th way that the deck is stacked against the complainant: secrecy!***

The whole process of how the TMB operates and how it uses the expert opinions that it depends on to make decisions is secret. At one point I had been trying for more than 5 months to extract a few answers about the process from the Director of the TMB without receiving any response. Finally, I received an email from the executive secretary of the TMB asking that I resend the letter requesting information because it seemed to be lost. I had sent the original letter by certified mail 5 months before, so I am certain that the Director's office received my questions. I had even tried to get the Office of the Governor of the State of Texas to write a letter encouraging an answer, and the governor's office had refused to get involved. ***How many Texas taxpayers know that tax money goes to support a secret process that is supposed to look out for them but does nothing more than protect bad doctors?***

I am by no means the only one to suspect that the TMB is failing miserably in its mission of protecting the citizens of Texas from bad doctors. In a column in the *Houston Chronicle* on December 30, 2004, entitled "License to kill," the author admonished the TSBME that it had better end the medical career of Dr. Eric Scheffey when it deliberated on his case in February 2005. According to the writer, this doctor performed many unnecessary operations and when he operated he often made mistakes, resulting in the deaths of at least 4 people. His insurers have paid out more than $10 million in claims to his victims. The editorial asserts, "As bad as Scheffey's incompetence and conscienceless behavior is, [is also] that of the doctors and hospitals who enabled Scheffey to continue practicing, knowing the high price paid by his patients...*Even after warnings and other disciplinary action—even after Scheffey was arrested driving a car containing cocaine and admitted that he used cocaine for at least 18 months, the [Texas Medical] board elected to put him on probation rather than pulling his license.*" In fact on February 4, 2005, the TMB did revoke the doctor's license, and after an appeal it became final on March 18, 2005; however, according to the TMB website posting on this physician (accessed 2/11/06), the revocation of his license is under appeal with the 126th Court in Travis County, Texas. The TMB information posted on this physician suggests that he may still have privileges at 2 hospitals in Pasadena, Texas. I recommend that you access the TMB website and see how long it takes you to determine the exact status of Scheffey's medical license. *You might want to note that Scheffey's initial license revocation, which was stayed, occurred in 1986, presumably before he killed any patients!*

I cannot understand why a physician with a record such as Scheffey's is not in jail for armed robbery; then it would not matter whether he had a medical license or not. When a physician does unnecessary surgery he is acting no differently than a thug who threatens a woman on the street with a loaded gun, and then steals her money. The threat the physician points at the patient is that the surgery or an invasive procedure is essential to the patient's recovery of health, and this makes the patient fearful of failing to comply, just as the gun does in a street robbery. The motives of the physician doing unnecessary surgery are exactly the same as those of the street robber: he wants money without giving anything of value in return, and he is willing to risk another's life to get it. *A new concept needs to be developed in the minds of police investigators and prosecuting attorneys, that of the "physician armed robber."* Later, I will discuss changes in the law that would encourage this type of prosecution to protect patients from unnecessary, and often risky, cutting on their bodies.

After I exhausted my appeals process with the TMB, I sent a certified letter to the director of the TMB on May 16, 2005, asking a number of questions about their processes and how they handled my son's case specifically. Much later, I followed this up with faxes and emails until apparently the TMB deduced that I was not going to go away. Here I list some of those questions and the TMB responses, which I finally received on January 16, 2006, 8 months later. This will give you insight into the attitudes of the director concerning the way he ran the board and how responsive he was to citizen inquiry. Besides the secrecy of the process and composition and activities of the DPRC, I was interested in the continuing medical education (CME) requirements in Texas and enforcement of those requirements.

1) What is the basis for requiring secrecy in your processes? Answer: "All board investigative files are statutorily confidential as provided by Sec. 164.007 of the Medical Practice Act.

2) Why is the DPRC composed mostly of physicians? Answer: "The overall board membership is determined by statute, specifically Sec. 152.003 of the Medical Practice Act. Sec. 152.003 provides that the board consists of nineteen members, seven of whom are public members."

3) What is the basis of always having an "expert" physician in the critical path to disciplining a physician? Answer: None given to me.

4) How did the DPRC handle the 3 ethical issues I raised [lack of informed consent, no written recommendations to the victim, and falsification of the medical records]? Answer: That's a secret we keep from you.

5) How many times has the DPRC disciplined a physician for failing to provide informed consent? Answer: An answer would require "depletion of agency resources." In other words we are too lazy.

6) How many times has the DPRC disciplined a physician for falsifying medical records? Answer: An answer would require "depletion of agency resources." Again, we are too lazy.

7) What percentage of CME submissions [required of doctors to show that they have taken continuing medical education] are reviewed each year? Answer: 1%.

8) After my complaint did you investigate the CME of the older cardiologist or consulting cardiologist? Answer. That's a secret we keep from you.

9) Did you investigate my allegation that Dr. PIT falsified her medical records? Answer. That's a secret we keep from you.

10) Can you explain to me how ignoring the clinical practice guideline for potassium replacement by my son's cardiologists is consistent with care that exceeded medical standards as asserted by your last expert? Answer: None given to me.

11) Were your "experts" given a copy of my complaint to review? Answer. None given to me.

An 8-page letter dated January 25, 2006, was sent from the legal counsel of the TMB to the Chief, Open Records Division of the Office of the Attorney General of Texas. I received a copy of that letter, whose purpose was to show the attorney general that I should not be given any more information by the TMB. I'd like to highlight one observation from that letter. Quote: "The confidentiality of this information [expert reports] is crucial to the mission of this agency. The [Texas Medical] Board is charged with the responsibility to protect the public by disciplinary action against licensees. Public disclosure of investigative information would hinder any investigation. If those providing expert reports believed their statements could be made public, they might not be as responsive or candid. Equally important, the Board would find it more difficult to recruit expert physician reviewers. Physicians are very concerned about potential lawsuits when they render a medical opinion. The fact that the State can afford to pay only a fraction of the going rate for expert opinions makes the concern of being sued far outweigh the financial remuneration." *This is TMB bureaucratic bunk!* A report by the Institute of Medicine (IOM) report (2001) cites evidence from 4 studies suggesting that "open disclosure of errors may *decrease* the likelihood of malpractice loss." The emphasis is the IOM's.

In my field of science research, papers receive review by a process that keeps the identity of the reviewer secret, but conveys to the author the exact wording of the reviewer's findings. To my knowledge no scientific journal pays any of its expert reviewers for reviewing a manuscript; scientists accept this responsibility as part of being a scientist. In fact, when I review another scientist's manuscript I am more thorough and balanced than I would be if it all were going to be kept secret. If I have to be harsh on the manuscript, then it is reassuring for me to know that the author will see my suggestions but never know my identity. The TMB needs to wake up to this reality and cease hiding its so-called expert opinions behind a wall of secrecy. *Complainants do not want the expert's identity, only their written "expert" opinion, which I suspect is shallow and uninformed in most cases because there is no accountability or quality control,*

and because physicians are extremely reluctant to hold each other accountable for fatal errors.

Separately, a TMB investigator has told me that physician experts are paid only $100 per hour for their reviews, which is consistent with the letter to the attorney general. I do not believe the fundamental problem of the TMB's secretive approach is going to be changed by paying more money to each expert. They portray this as a trade-off between fear of being sued and remuneration. Visibility of the opinions would improve the quality of expert reviews, especially if the expert is required to discuss the records in terms of clinical practice guidelines (CPGs), informed consent, evidence-based medicine, and consistency of the records. ***Why not make it part of practicing medicine in Texas to require that each licensed physician participate in the expert review process?*** If you want to be licensed in the state, then you will participate by giving up to 8 hours per year of expert opinion to the TMB. This could even count toward your CME requirement. The ultimate solution would be to mix "Maintenance of Certification" testing and records from malpractice allegations, but blind the expert to the source of the records (more on this in Chapter 10). Your identity, but not your opinion, would be kept secret, and you might actually learn some things that would improve your own practice, that is increase the safety of your own patients.

The Department of Health and Human Services in Inaction

The DHHS backs the clinic where my son had his last visit with any physician (the PIT doctor) and I had a hope that I could get some truth by asking a branch of the federal government, supported by all our tax dollars, to investigate. My main concern with that clinic visit was the false statement the PIT had placed in the record that my son and his parents refused a pacemaker and that an electroencephalogram was recommended and refused. It took many calls into the federal bureaucracy to determine whose job it was to investigate claims such as mine. On March 10, 2004, I sent a letter to the Associate Administrator for Primary Health Care of the Bureau of Primary Health Care of the Department of Health and Human Services. In my letter, which included enclosures of information I had sent to the director of the clinic "backed" by the federal government, I made it clear that a physician working in one of their clinics had falsified her medical records pertaining to my son's office visit.

In a letter dated April 22, 2004, from the above individual, a physician, he stated that he would "obtain and review additional information regarding this matter. This process will take some time to ensure a careful and comprehensive assessment." Many months and phone calls later, I received a letter dated October 4, 2004, stating that "As part of our quality assurance process, we carefully reviewed the information available to address your concerns regarding misconduct from a doctor employed by one of our grantees. We did not find evidence to support your allegation that Dr. PIT willfully recorded false information in your son's medical record. I apologize for the delay in responding." I sent back a reply to the agency physician asking the extent to which he had investigated my allegations of falsifying information. *In mid-December I received a reply, again apologizing for the delay in response, and stating that the investigation was closed.*

At that time I assumed I had exhausted my efforts to get any truth out of the federal government, but some months later I decided to lodge a Freedom of Information Act (FOIA) request to see if I could discover whether their investigation had any substance to it. Was there any hope that I might find out the truth? On May 22, 2005, I filed a FOIA request with the agency that handles these matters in Bethesda, Maryland. I agreed to pay for any cost to the federal government associated with my request. In response to my request, the agency sent me a highly censored summary of some cardiologist's rehash of my son's medical records. It contained no indication that anyone had actually investigated my claim that the records at the grantee clinic were falsified. *One statement that got past the censor's knife was this: "Two further details to make note of. Dr. PIT's dictated report from Mr. James visit at the [clinic] has no documentation as to when it was dictated or transcribed."* I assume the second detail was censured. I knew from a phone conversation I had with a computer operator at that clinic that they had had a state-of-the-art medical records system since the early 1990s, and that it places date stamps on all records and archives the times of any changes. I have confirmed this information by visiting the website of the clinic. It brags copiously about the leadership the clinic has shown in using electronic medical records since the mid-1990s. I had asked the DHHS for an investigation of record falsification, not another cardiologist's opinion.

I wasn't yet finished with the "feds." On June 19, 2005, I appealed the FOIA response and asked that the case be reopened and that they actually go find out whether my son's medical records had been modified by the PIT after his death. After many more calls to determine the status of my appeal, I received a letter on October 14, 2005, lamenting the reorganizations that were underway, but finally assigning my appeal to a specific person. After I had made more nagging calls, I received a letter from a Deputy Assistant Secretary for Public Affairs. This person asserted that "This review [done by the DHHS] addressed the quality of the medical care provided and whether the medical records were incorrectly edited." She included the statement bolded above as one of the enclosures to her letter. *I can only scream in amazement and protest as to how the DHHS determined that my son's medical records were not "incorrectly edited" when they cannot even tell when they were "dictated or transcribed." I suppose they took the word of the accused PIT that she did nothing wrong!* Despite the DHHS's idiotic and secretive approach to investigating my allegations of falsifying of medical records, I was able to glean an interesting observation from the copies of Alex's medical records that they sent me. It comes from the hand of the older cardiologist in the form of a surprising new document that had not been part of Alex's records before (Exhibit 12).

Near the top of his new "consultation report" it is stated, "This chart is being dictated on 09/08/2003 to fulfill requirements for dictation in Medical Records on a previously admitted patient." *This is more than 1 year after the older cardiologist evaluated my son and almost one year after he died.* I wonder whose requirements he is fulfilling. He reports on Alex's ECG, as if there had been just one: "sinus bradycardia with nonspecific T-wave inversion in leads 2, 3, and AVF." *This is an utterly unprofessional observation and ignores the profound importance of my son's 479 ms QTc printed on the ECG and his PVCs.* The most striking T-wave inversion was in V4, as shown in Exhibit 4, and leads aVL, V3, V5, and V6 also showed T-wave inversions; trace V2 did *not* show T-wave inversions.

Here's the older cardiologist's belated formal assessment: "I think this gentleman [referring to Alex] had an episode of exercise-induced syncope of unclear etiology. We obviously need to rule out cardiac etiologies as well as metabolic and possible neurologic evaluation." *This is crass backfill by the older cardiologist. He never suspected a metabolic or neurologic etiology for my son's syncope until long after Alex was dead. And he certainly never proposed any strategy to pursue a metabolic or neurological cause.* The physician progress record on my son clearly shows that he never had these thoughts at the time. His recommendations in his belated report followed: "We will obtain an exercise treadmill test to test maximum heart rate to see if we can reproduce this [syncope?] as well as a baseline echocardiogram and go from there. I would like to arrange from electrophysiology consultants to evaluate him as well." This shows clearly that this older cardiologist was focused exclusively on a cardiac cause for my son's syncope. Why did he not call a neurologist if he was concerned about a neurological cause? This document shows at the bottom that it was dictated on "03/08/04," exactly 6 months after 09/08/2003, when the opening statement asserted that it was being dictated. This pathetic

John T. James, Ph.D

record is nothing more than the older cardiologist's sloppy attempt to put
a band-aid on top of an infected shotgun wound.

NAME: JAMES, ALEX MR#000535093
PHYSICIAN: <deleted> LOCATION:
ADMISSION DATE: 08/19/02 DISCHARGE DATE: 08/22/02

CONSULTATION REPORT:

ABDOMEN:	No hepatosplenomegaly or tenderness.
EXTREMETIES:	Good pulses. No cyanosis, clubbing, or edema.
ELECTROCARDIOGRAM:	Sinus bradycardia with nonspecific T-wave inversion in leads 2, 3, and AVF.

ASSESSMENT:

I THINK THIS GENTLEMAN HAD AN EPISODE OF EXERCISE INDUCED
SYNCOPE OF UNCLEAR ETIOLOGY. WE OBVIOUSLY NEED TO RULE
OUT CARDIAC ETIOLOGIES AS WELL AS METABOLIC DISTURBANCES
AND POSSIBLE NEUROLOGIC EVALUATION.

RECOMMENDATIONS:

We will obtain an exercise treadmill test to maximum heart rate to see if we can
reproduce this as well as a baseline echocardiogram and go from there. I would
like to arrange from electrophysiology consultants to evaluate him as well.

Exhibit 12. Late entry into Alex's medical record by the older cardiologist.

Chapter 7
To Err Is Human, to Ignore Errors Unconscionable

Warnings from the Past

Everyone makes errors while performing their job; there are no exceptions. In most professions errors do not result in death. In medicine, mistakes by physicians often cause "iatrogenic" disease or death. Although physicians control most aspects of the health delivery system, it would be unfair to blame them for all the lethal medical errors made; however, some studies have specifically targeted the physicians' *direct* role in making such catastrophic mistakes. An article published in *JAMA*, and authored by 4 physicians from the Harvard Medical School, was called "Incidence and characteristics of preventable iatrogenic cardiac arrests" (Bedell et al., 1991). The authors studied a group of 203 patients who experienced cardiac arrest in a university teaching hospital in 1981 and on whom resuscitation was attempted. Of that group of cardiac arrests, 14% were due to an iatrogenic event. Those events included medication errors (44%) and inadequate response (28%) by physicians to clinical signs and symptoms such as dyspnea (difficulty breathing) and tachypnea (very rapid breathing) in the patients. Sixty-one percent of these patients who had cardiac arrests died.

Medication errors may have actually increased in frequency since the early 1980s. According to death certificate data, which can have significant limitations, the number of medication errors climbed from about 2,900 in 1983 to 7,400 in 1993 (Phillips et al., 1998). In a later article authored by 10 physicians, a Ph.D, and a doctor of pharmacy (Pharm.D.), entitled "Medication errors in acute cardiac care" (Freedman et al., 2002), the authors note that "an ***important issue in acute cardiac care is failure to follow guidelines by omitting medications demonstrated to be effective*.**" The authors cite other studies showing that a major percentage of myocardial infarct patients are not given aspirin soon after admission. Conversely, the authors report that: "despite previous educational efforts, drugs withdrawn from the market due to major adverse outcomes associated with their use, continued to be prescribed inappropriately." The authors conclude that "the problem of medication errors must be introduced to health professionals early in their training and the principles reinforced repeatedly." In other words, there is a lot of educational work to be done before medication errors are properly controlled.

In the turbulent years that marked our involvement in the Vietnam War, I wanted to be a physician. During that time I gathered a collection of books related to medicine. From that collection I still have a now yellow-brown-paged paperback called "The American Medical Machine," written by Senator Abraham Ribicoff in 1972. After listing a number of instances of doctors failing to police their ranks, Sen. Ribicoff stated that "*the lesson of all of this is that medicine is far too important to be left to the doctors…That [observation] also means some drastic improvements [are needed] in the mechanisms for finding, controlling, and disciplining incompetent doctors*." He further stated, in a prophetic statement, "More specifically, our efforts are an attempt to establish as clearly as possible the following proposition: to receive medical care is the right; to provide it the privilege. In a fundamental sense, that is the only real issue in medicine. That is all that medicine is about or should have been about. That is all it should ever be about. Unless this country can accept the undiluted truth of this statement and make it the basis for national policy and national action, we are likely to face a much more severe version of what we have come to call 'the health care crisis' for the rest of this century and well into the next." One might now ask, "How were we as a nation doing at the end of the century?"

As the New Millennium Begins

A troubling answer to that question can be gleaned from *To Err Is Human, Building a Safer Health Care System*, a book written by the Committee on Quality of Health Care in America of the Institute of Medicine (IOM), and published by the National Academy Press in 2000. The committee consisted of CEOs of several large corporations, CEOs of health care providers, and clinicians from several medical schools.

What did this esteemed committee deduce about our health care system? They estimated that in 1997 between 44,000 and 98,000 Americans died as a result of medical errors made during hospitalization. Their estimate was based on 2 studies that set a high bar for definition of a medical mistake, including concurrence from 2 reviewers that an error had occurred and that only errors documented in the medical record were considered. Apparently, my son's death would not have been counted as an error in this system because several cardiologists have said his care met or exceeded the standard. *Even if the IOM's lower estimate were used, this is more people dying each year from medical errors than from motor vehicle accidents, breast cancer, or AIDS.* The authors went on to conclude, "The goal of this report is to break the cycle of inaction. The status quo is not acceptable and cannot be tolerated any longer. Despite the cost pressures, liability constraints, resistance to change and other seemingly insurmountable barriers, it is simply not acceptable for patients to be harmed by the same health care system that is supposed to offer healing and comfort...The combined goal of the recommendations is for the external environment to create sufficient pressure to make errors costly to health care organizations and providers, so they are compelled to take action to improve safety. At the same time, there is a need to enhance knowledge and tools to improve safety and break down legal and cultural barriers that impede safety improvement."

The IOM report deals with many aspects of the health care industry that should be targeted for improvement and government oversight. One recommendation that parallels the thesis of this book is this: "Performance standards and expectations for health professionals should focus greater attention on patient safety. *Health professional licensing bodies should (1) implement periodic re-examinations and re-licensing of doctors, nurses, and other key providers, based on both competence and knowledge of safety practices; and (2) work with certifying and credentialing organizations to develop more effective methods to identify unsafe providers and take action.*"

The report considers the economic costs of medication-related errors alone and concludes from a study of such errors in 2 "prestigious teaching hospitals" that "If these findings are generalizable, the increased hospital costs alone of preventable adverse drug events affecting in-patients are about $2 billion [each year] for the nation as a whole. These figures offer only a very modest estimate of the economic magnitude of the problem since hospital patients represent only a small portion of the total population at risk, and direct hospital costs are only a fraction of total costs." The report examines another aspect of our costly health care system and concludes, "*Purchasers and patients pay for errors when insurance costs and co-payments are inflated by services that would not have been necessary had proper care been provided.* It is impossible for the nation to achieve the greatest value possible from the billions of dollars spent on medical care if the care contains errors."

In an interesting article in *JAMA* entitled "Is US health really the best in the world?," a physician from Johns Hopkins School of Hygiene and Public Health conveys a sobering answer to her question (Starfield, 2000): "the US population does not have anywhere near the best health in the world." She cites studies showing that 20 to 30% of U.S. patients receive contraindicated care and that of 13 developed countries studied, the U.S. ranks on average next to last in a variety of quality of health care indicators. She mentions the findings reported by the IOM (2000) that as many as 98,000 Americans die each year as a result of medical errors in hospitals. This estimate was based on chart reviews, which are known to understate the actual level of injury by several times (Brennan et al, 2005). To this she would add 80,000 deaths for hospital-acquired infections and another 106,000 deaths from adverse reactions to drugs given as indicated (Lazarou et al., 1998). Her final estimate for iatrogenic deaths ranged from 225,000 to 284,000 human beings per year. These estimates were derived mostly from data on hospitalized patients. One study she cites on outpatient care estimated that 199,000 additional deaths result each year from adverse medical effects occurring in outpatients (Weingart et al., 2000). Death rates in the range of 300,000+ per year place iatrogenic death in third place of all causes of death, behind heart disease (685,000) and all cancers (557,000) and well ahead of cerebral-vascular disease (158,000) and chronic lung disease (126,000). To these frightening estimates one could add the 100,000 heart failure patients who die early because they did not receive beta blockers as they should have (Gheorghiade et al., 2002). In late 2005 Dr. Starfield wrote a less technical article for the lay public in which she makes frightening observations about our health care system and proposes some changes: http://bostonreview.net/BR30.6/starfield.html (accessed 11/21/2006).

The World Health Organization (http://www.who.int/inf-pr-2000/en/pr2000-life.html) released what they call "healthy life expectancy" rankings showing the U.S. ranked 24th. At that Web address, Christopher Murray, M.D., Ph.D., Director of WHO's Global Programme on Evidence for Health Policy, states, ***"Basically, you die earlier and spend more time disabled if you're an American rather than a member of most other advanced countries."***

I have many middle-aged friends who believe they have received error-laden medical care from physicians, but in most cases they have eventually found a competent, attentive physician who has been able to diagnose and treat their illness. Once that happens, the error-laden care is forgotten and the person continues with their life, and the poorly-performing physicians are never held accountable for their mistakes. My observation is borne out by another conclusion of the IOM regarding medical mistakes. Referring to such mistakes, they wrote, ***"Silence surrounds this issue [of medical errors]. For the most part, consumers believe they are protected. Media coverage has been limited to reporting of anecdotal cases. Licensure and accreditation confer, in the eyes of the public, 'Good Housekeeping Seal of Approval.' Yet, licensing and accreditation processes have focused*** *only limited attention on the issue [of physician incompetence], and even those minimal efforts have confronted some resistance from health care organizations and providers.*" Later in the IOM book the experts stated, "The most important barrier to improving patient safety is lack of awareness of the extent to which errors occur daily in all health care settings and organizations. *This lack of awareness exists because the vast majority of errors are not reported, and they are not reported because personnel fear they will be punished.*"

A recent editorial by a physician entitled "Who said medicine means never having to say you're sorry?" (Matheson, 2006) contains a number of noteworthy statements, including "Everyone makes mistakes. So, why do we doctors have such difficulty admitting that?" He lists a number of possibilities: it's hard to admit error and apologize, it connotes weakness, it invites legal worries, and physicians have narcissistic tendencies. He states, "I've found that physicians rarely receive admonition well and tend, as a whole, to be defensive. This can ring true in a hospital setting, where questions can be perceived as threatening or undermining." He points out that "studies show that improved physician-patient relations help diminish malpractice lawsuits." This voice from the "inside" is refreshing to hear. I think in a back-door sort of way, responsible physicians are pleading with us patients to do something. *Physicians are not going to consistently criticize and regulate individuals within their professional community; the control must come from outside.*

One additional problem that bears on my son's death is that he received highly compartmentalized and uncoordinated care at 3 medical institutions. This is a recipe for mistakes, and the IOM seems to agree. Their report asserted, "The decentralized and fragmented nature of the health care delivery system (some would say 'non-system') also contributes to unsafe conditions, and serves as an impediment to efforts to improve [patient] safety...*Unsafe care is one of the prices we pay for not having organized systems of care with clear lines of accountability.*" In the case of my son's death, there will always be questions about who was in charge. Was it the attending physician, was it the older cardiologist, or was it the consultant cardiologist?

Ongoing Danger to Patients

One would like to imagine that the IOM report of 2000 is now history and that the health care system in this country has made dramatic improvements in response to the criticisms leveled at it by the report. Unfortunately, that is far from the case. In a report called "Five Years After 'To Err Is Human'" published in *JAMA*, 2 physicians (Leape and Berwick, 2005) summarized the state of progress. They wrote, "Small but consequential changes have gradually spread through hospitals, due largely to concerted activities by hospital associations, professional societies, and accrediting bodies.... Although these efforts are affecting safety at the margin, their overall impact is hard to see in national statistics; little evidence exists from any source that systematic improvements in [patient] safety are widely available." The authors concluded, "In sum, the groundwork for improving safety has been laid these past 5 years, but progress is frustratingly slow. Building a culture of safety is proving to be an immense task and the barriers are formidable. Whether significant progress will be achieved in the next 5 years depends on how successfully those barriers are addressed...*If the experience of the past 5 years demonstrates anything, it is that neither strong evidence of ongoing serious harm nor the activities, examples, and progress of a courageous minority are sufficient to generate the national commitment needed to rapidly advance patient safety. Such a commitment is not likely to be forthcoming without more sustained and powerful pressure on hospital boards and leaders—pressure that must come from outside the health industry.*"

In another article in *JAMA* discussing the status of patient safety in hospitals since the IOM report, the conclusion is equally unsettling. The authors looked at seven variables, designed to represent the most important patient safety measures, in more than 100 hospitals in 2002 and again in 2004 (Longo et al., 2005). The authors concluded, "The current status of hospital patient safety systems is not close to meeting IOM recommendations. *Data are consistent with recent reports that patient safety system progress is slow and is a cause for great concern.* Efforts for improvement must be accelerated."

One must ask if it is possible that our medical care system in the United States is simply the best it can be and that other developed nations experience the same magnitude of errors in patient care. *The answer to that is that the U.S. stands out among developed nations for inefficient, error-laden health care that is difficult to access and too costly.* An article in the journal *Health Affairs* entitled "Taking the Pulse of Health Care Systems: Experiences of Patients with Health Problems in Six Countries" and written by a group of 7 experts in research and health delivery systems characterizes the experiences of seriously ill patients in Australia, Canada, Germany, New Zealand, the United Kingdom, and the United States (Schoen et al., 2005). The study involved between 700 and 1,800 patients from each country. The percentage of patients reporting that a medical mistake was made in their treatment or care, or that the wrong medication or dose was given, was between 17 and 19%, except for the United States, where the percentage was 22%. Among those patients reporting that they had been given incorrect results for a diagnostic or lab test, the percentages ranged from 3 to 7% in all countries except the U.S., where the percentage was 10%. One must remember that these data come from patients who discover that their health care provider has made an error. As I have shown previously, most patients are unaware when errors are made in their health care, so these percentages and the position of the United States among them are alarming.

Two physicians and a doctor of pharmacology make a number of troubling observations about the care of patients with heart failure in this country in an article entitled "Treatment gaps in the management of heart failure" (Gheorghiade et al., 2002) in *Reviews in Cardiovascular Medicine*. They cite a "crude analysis" of the epidemiology of the 287,000 Americans who died of heart failure in the United States in 1999. Of those, about 100,000 could have been saved with beta-blocker therapy. This observation was made from data available at the time from the American Heart Association and clinical trials of beta-blockers, showing a 35% success rate in life-saving treatment. Here is one of the authors' main points: ***Despite conclusive data supporting their benefits, only 20-40% of patients with heart failure are treated with beta-blockers.*** They advocate a 2-step process in which, firstly, barriers to the implementation of evidence-based medicine must be identified, and then those barriers must be overcome.

We still find tremendous room for improvement in the care of cardiac patients in the U.S. This observation comes from an article entitled "Adherence to heart failure quality-of-care indicators in U.S. hospitals," published in the *Archives of Internal Medicine* (Farnow et al., 2005). The authors looked at conformity to 4 indicators of core performance measures promulgated by the Joint Commission on Accreditation of Healthcare Organizations (JCAHO) for care of heart failure (HF) in more than 81,000 patients admitted to hospitals from July 1, 2002 through December 31, 2003. These were the 4 indicators: HF1: proportion of patients given complete *written* instructions on activity level, diet, medications, follow-up appointment, and what to do if symptoms worsen, HF2: portion of patients who received appropriate assessment of left ventricle function, HF3: portion of patients who should have been and were prescribed ACE (acetylcholinesterase) inhibitors, and HF4: portion of patients who had a history of smoking and were given smoking cessation advice during the hospital stay. The median rates of conformity are shown in the table below for academic and non-academic hospitals.

The authors cite a study that used performance rates for the equivalent of HF2 and HF3 in 1998-1999 before the performance indicators were adopted by JCAHO. In 1998 to 1999, the equivalent of HF2 was 66% and the equivalent of HF3 was 72%, suggesting that patients are now getting more measurements of their ventricular function, but no improvement in their rate of prescription of ACE inhibitors (my conclusion). It also seems that the non-academic hospital where Alex received his EP test was among the 68% of reported hospitals that fail to give written instructions on activity levels. The authors concluded, *"The continued persistence of suboptimal compliance with these measures [of cardiac patient care] and the significant variability between hospitals in this compliance and in outcome variables provides a compelling rationale for implementation of new systems to improve hospital performance."*

Variable number	Indicator	Academic hospitals	Non-academic hospitals
HF1	Given written instructions	12 %	32 %
HF2	Measure left ventricle function	88 %	85 %
HF3	Prescribe ACE inhibitors	75 %	71 %
HF4	Advice on smoking cessation	36 %	45 %

Table 2. Median compliance with quality-of-care indicators in cardiac patients, 2002-2003.

The excess death rate in hospitals is sufficiently alarming that the Institute for Healthcare Improvement launched an effort called the "100,000 Lives Campaign" in late 2004. Their intention was to identify 100,000 patients by June 2006 who had been discharged from hospitals and who, absent the changes achieved during the campaign, would have left the hospital dead (Berwick et al., 2006). The campaign was based on 6 "highly feasible" interventions for which efficacy is documented in the peer-reviewed literature and reflected in standards set by relevant specialty societies and government agencies. One of the key interventions was evidence-based care for acute myocardial infarctions. This would include the use of aspirin, beta-blockers, ACE inhibitors, and timely reperfusion, and smoking cessation. By the middle of 2006, Dr. Berwick was claiming that 122,300 lives had been saved in participating hospitals during the 18-

month period, and this received much attention in the press. Unfortunately, the estimate of 122,300 was derived from an apparent measured reduction of 33,000 deaths. The methods used for the "conversion" to 122,300 from 33,000 may not be robust (Wollschlaeger, 2006). I have not yet seen a peer-reviewed publication attesting to Dr. Berwick's numerical success.

Recently some surprising findings have come from physicians deeply concerned with the lack of quality patient care in the American medical system. Some writers have suggested that the worst medical care is given to the poorest, uninsured Americans who do not have easy access to the medical system. This seems to fit with what we would intuitively expect; however, this idea is not true, according to recent findings. *Americans, regardless of gender, age, race, education, income, and health insurance all receive uniformly poor medical care as measured by whether that care followed quality-of-care scores widely recognized for 30 chronic and acute health problems.* In an article published in the *New England Journal of Medicine*, a team of 7 investigators, including 3 physicians, used medical records from 6700 people living in 12 communities to determine the quality of care they received from their health care system (Asch et al., 2006). On average, participants received 55% of the care they should have had. The recommended care was based on indicators of quality selected by medical experts from those established in RAND's Quality Assessment Tools database. The types of care were broken down into the categories of acute care, chronic care, and preventive care. Across these 3 categories and for all groups listed above, the care never got better than 61% and never worse than 50%. Thus, if you have choices in where you seek medical care and you have insurance, you should not necessarily expect recommended care much more than half the time. The authors of this article state, "These results underscore the profound and systemic nature of the quality-of-care problem."

Another recent study has shown that not receiving treatment consistent with quality-of-care indicators is a risk factor for premature death in older patients. In an article entitled "Quality of care is associated with survival in vulnerable older patients," a team of 13 medical specialists, mostly physicians, looked at survival over 3 years in patients over 65 who were enrolled in managed care organizations in 1998 and 1999 (Higashi et al., 2005). They used quality-of-care indicators for 21 different clinical conditions and divided the patients into 2 equal-sized groups: those receiving above the average score on quality-of-care indicators and those receiving a below-average score; the average quality score was only 53%. In the 2 groups starting the study (186 in each group), the number of deaths was the same in the first 400 days; however, after 1000 days, 28 were dead in the group with quality scores above 53% and 49 were dead in the group with quality scores below 53%. The authors stopped short of stating that better compliance of health care providers with quality-of-care recommendations saves lives. They concluded, "Better performance on process quality measures is strongly associated with better survival among community-dwelling vulnerable older adults." An editorial follow-up to this study (Williams, 2005) discussed the process problems that the team above uncovered and stated: *"Another part of the problem is the way clinicians use, or don't use, existing medical knowledge to care for patients.* None of us knows everything. Even when we know enough, we may be rushed or tired or distracted or we may not have the right resources to do the best job possible."

The results of a study of outpatient care gathered from 1992 to 2002 on persons who need lipid-lowering drugs to manage their risk of coronary artery disease are troubling (Ma et al., 2005). The authors assert that "evidence-based practice guidelines focus on low-density lipoprotein cholesterol (LDL-C) as the primary risk reduction therapy …[and that that] therapy should be adjusted to individual absolute risk for coronary heart disease." There are 3 categories of risk, and those in the highest risk group or whose risk cannot be managed by lifestyle changes, should be given statin drug therapy. The authors report a trend to increasing use of statins (from 10% in 1992 to 50% in 2000) in the patients with high concentrations of cholesterol in their blood, and then they identify a number of causes of the low therapeutic rate, including lack of physician awareness of the guideline. They comment that "despite notable improvements in the past decade, clinical practice fails to institute recommended statin therapy during many ambulatory visits of patients at moderate-to-high cardiovascular risk."

Treatment of heart attacks is still an active area of research. A recent article in *JAMA* (Alexander et al., 2005) reported, from a survey of more than 30,000 heart attack victims in nearly 400 hospitals, that 42 percent of the patients received doses of blood thinners outside the recommended range. This resulted in a 30 percent increased chance of major bleeding compared to those given the correct dose of anticoagulants. The death rate was higher among patients given excessive doses.

A major finding has been reported for care of patients with stable coronary artery disease that you should know about (Boden, et al. 2007). The study was published in the highly-respected *New England Journal of Medicine,* and I counted 23 authors, the vast majority of them physicians (Boden et al., 2007). The authors note that in the United States 1 million coronary-artery-stent procedures were performed in 2004. Based on another study, approximately 85% of these were in patients with stable coronary artery disease. The stent procedure involves entering one or more of the patient's partially-obstructed coronary arteries and inserting a metal device that expands to open the lumen of the partially blocked artery. They also note that treatment guidelines from 2002 (Gibbons, et al., 2003) for patients with stable coronary artery disease *do not* call for use of stents as an initial treatment. Initial treatment should be with optimal medical therapy, which includes risk factor reduction, lifestyle changes, and medication. The authors basically address the question: do the patients with stable coronary artery disease who receive coronary artery stents and optimal medical therapy experience a reduced risk of death or myocardial infarction over the next 5 years compared to those receiving only optimal medical therapy? In other words, are the guidelines correct to specify optimal medical therapy alone as an initial treatment?

A selected population of 2287 patients with stable coronary artery disease was randomly assigned to one of 2 groups. Both groups received optimal medical therapy; however, only one group received a stent procedure. The investigators concluded that the stent therapy *did not* reduce the risk of death or myocardial infarction when added to optimal medical therapy. Their findings showed that existing guidelines are correct; the stent procedure can be safely deferred in patients with stable coronary artery disease, provided that optimal medical therapy is instituted and maintained. I noticed that there were 35 periprocedural (iatrogenic) heart attacks in the stent group, which means that the attempt to place a stent caused a heart attack

In an associated editorial two physicians (Hochman and Steg, 2007) note that substantial health care cost savings can be expected because of the findings reported by Boden et al. (2007).You may have the same question I did. Why in the heck were cardiologists doing so many expensive and risky stent procedures in 2004 when guidelines for initial care of patients with stable coronary artery disease did *not* call for this procedure? I think we both suspect the answer to that question. If you estimate the number of stable patients receiving this procedure each year (at least 50% of 1 million, or 500,000) and multiply that by the typical $50,000 per procedure (range from my insurance company $26,200 to $84,400), the product is 25 *billion* dollars! If your cardiologist proposes to put a stent in your coronary arteries, ask him if he is following guidelines from the American College of Cardiology and the American Heart Association. If he looks at you like he does not know what you are talking about, find another cardiologist.

A book has just been published by a cardiologist in California advocating against many common invasive cardiac procedures. Dr. Howard

Wayne called his book "Do You Really Need Bypass Surgery? A Second Opinion." According to the book overview, "It provides an eye opening look at the coronary artery bypass surgery industry, and the cardiologists and surgeons who force bypass surgery, angioplasty, and stents on helpless, frightened patients who often have a benign heart problem, and even no symptoms...The author takes particular aim at what he considers the common and unethical practice of many cardiologists who use tactics he calls *medical terrorism*." Dr. Wayne is Director of the Noninvasive Heart Center in San Diego, California. He makes the point that cardiologists must sell 50-75 angiograms [left heart catheterizations] per year to patients to maintain hospital privileges. He claims remarkable success using optimal medical therapy for more than 2 decades. I like the title of an earlier book he wrote: "*How to Protect Your Heart from Your Doctor.*" You may want to investigate his website: http://www.heartprotect.com/the-books.shtml if your cardiologist recommends invasive procedures. I suspect Dr. Wayne is regarded as a heretic by those who make their lucrative living invading our hearts with their devices, and by those who manufacture such invasive devices.

In my opinion no one knows the extent to which poorly-performing physicians cause their patients to suffer and die. In the case of my son's death, a "team" of cardiologists was involved and 5 additional cardiologists have looked at his records and stated that he received care that met or exceeded medical standards. Yet, I trust that I have convinced you that his life could have been saved if he had been given electrolyte replacement therapy that was obviously needed based on a compelling diagnosis (acquired LQTS) and a nationally-established clinical guideline for potassium replacement. I also provided circumstantial data that a poorly performed catheterization caused injury of his ventricular septum, setting him up to die while he was running, an activity that he was warned against only while heavily sedated after an invasive test. Most publications dealing with the portion of physicians who are impaired for some reason suggest that this fraction is no more than a few percent. The sample of cardiologists who dealt with my son's records is by no means statistically rigorous; however, the fact that none of them saw his obvious diagnosis or knew about the medical guideline suggests that a large fraction of physicians calling themselves cardiologists have a tenuous grip on general knowledge in cardiology and on the guidelines that have been established to efficiently and safely treat patients.

To some extent my observation is supported by a recent report dealing with physicians in general. Two physicians, Leape and Fromson, (2006), began their report with the words, "*Physician performance failures are*

not rare and pose substantial threats to patient welfare and safety. Few hospitals respond to such failures promptly or effectively." The authors assert that hospitals must find better ways to monitor physician performance and seek remediation when required. They feel that a national effort is needed in this regard. In California the medical board estimated that 18% of physicians in that state abuse alcohol or drugs at some point in their career. The authors estimate that 4% of physicians have a problem with disruptive behavior and 10% demonstrate significant deficiencies in knowledge at some point in their career. I think this last estimate is misleading and far too low because the estimate was made from board examination failures, which tend to be taken when the examinee is full of knowledge after residency or a period of concerted study. I would argue that in general 10% of physicians may start out with insufficient knowledge in their specialty, but since there is no effective mechanism for them to recover general knowledge as they practice, this initial fraction is always lacking in general knowledge of their specialty. Furthermore, the percentage of uninformed physicians increases well above 10% as new knowledge enters the specialty and individual physicians never learn it. I believe this view is supported by the study that I describe below.

One would think that older, more experienced physicians would render better quality of care to their patients. The premise of an investigation by Choudhry et al. (2005) was that "Physicians with more experience are generally believed to have accumulated knowledge and skills during years in practice and therefore deliver high-quality care." The authors surveyed MEDLINE (the major database of medical research publications) for English-language reports, published from 1966 to 2004, of studies pertaining to this premise. Of 62 studies identified, 45 showed *decreasing* physician performance with increasing number of years in practice, 2 showed an initial increase and subsequent decline, 13 reported no association, and 2 reported increasing performance measures with increasing number of years in practice. The authors conclude, "***Physicians who have been in practice longer may be at risk for providing lower-quality care. Therefore, this subgroup of physicians may need quality improvement interventions***." In my opinion, this finding is not surprising because many physicians have no requirement to maintain knowledge and skills in their specialty.

As I finish summarizing the state of cardiology care in this country and look back on the causes of my son's death and the response of the accountability system to it, I realize that there really is not any meaningful standard of care for cardiology patients. Cardiologists see patients with stable coronary artery disease, heart failure or myocardial infarctions all the time and often do not get their treatment right. Why should I have ever expected cardiologists to recognize and treat the less common electrolyte depletion that my son had? ***The cardiologists' self-imposed standard of care is disassociated from guidelines and basic knowledge in cardiology. It is a myth; there is no standard. This statement does not in any way mean that there are not plenty of excellent cardiologists; it does mean there are far too many who lack the knowledge to effectively treat their patients, and some of these patients will die years before they should. Alex was one of them.***

Chapter 8
Who Says a Cardiologist Knows What He Is Doing?

Is Your Cardiologist a Cardiologist?

In general, physicians are licensed for the practice of medicine and not for a specific medical specialty such as cardiovascular disease. Thus, according to the IOM report (2001) called *Crossing the Quality Chasm: A New Health System for the 21st Century*, "Individual practitioners are thereby permitted [by licensure] to perform all activities that fall within medicine's broad scope of practice. Although a dermatologist would not likely perform open-heart surgery, doing so is not restricted by licensure." The report goes on to state, "Patients often seek out information about a physician's reputation and credentials." That's fine in principle, but in Texas at the time my son was being treated (or mistreated) by cardiologists there was no practical means of learning about the credentials of someone calling himself a cardiologist in Texas.

This all began to change in 2003; however, the resistance from physician groups remains steadfast. In an article in the May 5, 2003, issue of amednews.com—"The Newspaper for America's Physicians"— Damon Adams makes the following statement, "Physicians and medical societies object when a state proposes listing physician profiles and disciplinary actions on the Internet for consumer access. Doctors worry that medical board postings of malpractice information and disciplinary actions will scare away patients, supply attorneys with data for lawsuits and give the impression they are bad physicians." *This incredible attitude apparently voiced by some physicians demonstrates their arrogance. Basically, they believe their right to do unencumbered business as a physician supersedes the rights of patients to have some measure of the risk they are assuming by placing their trust in a specific physician.*

At this time it is possible to obtain considerable information about physicians in Texas through the TMB website, including their board certifications and training; however, how many Texans know that information is available? What does one do in situations like that of my son where he was delivered by ambulance to a specific hospital in an unfamiliar city? How bad does a physician have to be to receive some mark on his on-line record? I argued earlier that the TMB is so inept at disciplining physicians that the Web postings are nearly meaningless. Recently, I gave a talk about my son's care and mentioned my opinion of the TMB in disciplining physicians. A woman who had been involved with the TMB for years as a reporter said that I had gotten it right. Unless a physician is a flagrant alcohol or drug abuser, the TMB is not going to discipline them.

How Are Cardiologists Board Certified?

How much confidence should you place in a cardiologist because he is board certified? The American Board of Internal Medicine (ABIM) certifies cardiologists in the United States. A cardiologist must first be certified in internal medicine, and then certified in the subspecialty of "cardiovascular disease." The cardiologist can then be certified in an area of "added qualifications" such as "clinical cardiac electrophysiology" or "interventional cardiology." The ABIM defines requirements for specialists to maintain this certification; however, quoting from the ABIM website (accessed 4/29/05), "Internists and subspecialists certified in 1990 or later must complete the program to maintain certification. Everyone else [having life-time certification] is strongly urged to participate." *This means that a cardiologist who was certified as a specialist in cardiovascular disease before 1990 does not have to do anything to maintain ABIM certification!* Quoting again from the ABIM website, "In general, you do not need to maintain certification in internal medicine to recertify in a subspecialty.... Diplomats must have a valid certificate in cardiovascular disease to certify or recertify in the added qualifications of interventional cardiology and clinical cardiac electrophysiology." Thus, if you were certified in 1990 or later in cardiovascular disease, you do not have to maintain a general knowledge of internal medicine. The recertification cycle is 10 years long, so as of 2005, only those certified in cardiovascular disease between 1990 and 1995 have had to recertify their right to represent themselves as a board-certified cardiologist.

This observation about the system of specialty board certification may explain why my son's lead cardiologist knew so little cardiology. He failed to know the importance of a previous ECG that I offered to get from the Air Force, he failed to apply the widely-published medical standard for potassium replacement, and he failed to make the rather simple diagnosis of LQTS even though he knew and told me Alex's QTc was 480 ms. In his defense, the consultant he engaged also missed my son's obvious prolonged QT interval even after explicitly writing in his record that it was about 490 ms, and it seems that few cardiologists know to apply the guideline for potassium replacement. From publicly available information I have learned that this older "cardiologist" was board-certified in cardiovascular disease by the ABIM long before the 1990 adoption of maintenance of certification requirements. He had spent recent years engaged in practicing two demanding professions not related to cardiology. Was it any wonder he was not up on the latest guidelines and diagnostic procedures?

How Do Cardiologists Demonstrate Knowledge?

According to the ABIM website, the certification process has 3 facets: verification of credentials, completion of a Self-Evaluation Process, and completion of a secure exam in the area of expertise. The ABIM, in a kind letter to me dated August 18, 2005, provided me with the following statistics on persons certified in cardiovascular disease. Almost 22,000 physicians are certified in cardiovascular disease. More than half of these (53%) have lifetime certificates issued before 1990. The rest of the cardiologists (47%) hold 10-year limited certificates. Of the 53% with lifetime certification, only 2% participate in the "Maintenance of Certification (MOC)" voluntary program to demonstrate that their skills in cardiology are up to date. *This means that 52% of all active cardiologists have no intention of demonstrating to the ABIM that they are up to date in their knowledge and practice of cardiology. They have a lifetime certificate and that is all they need.* Of the 1% (2% of 53%) of lifetime-certified cardiologists who decided to voluntarily participate in the MOC, only 1/3rd have completed voluntary MOC. Of the cardiologists certified between 1990 and 1995, 93% have enrolled in MOC, and 83% (89% of the 93%) have completed MOC. The reason that 11% of those seeking MOC have not yet received it is that they have failed to complete the secure examination or one or more of the Self-Evaluation Process modules. I wonder if they are still calling themselves cardiologists.

The value of physician self-assessment has been called into question in a review article published recently in *JAMA* (Davis et al., 2006). The authors looked at a number of studies, involving physicians from developed countries, in which the self-assessment by those physicians could be compared to an external assessment. Of the 20 comparisons that qualified for the study, 13 showed little, no, or an inverse relationship between the measures. The other 7 comparisons showed positive associations. The authors concluded that "the preponderance of evidence suggests that physicians have limited ability to accurately self-assess. The process currently used to undertake professional development and evaluate competence may need to focus more on external assessment."

Physician specialty boards can have an important role in the movement toward improved patient care in the U.S.; however, they are going to have to listen more to patients and less to their physician constituency. Brennan et al. (2004) reported that a Gallup poll found that the public values board certification and maintenance of certification for physicians. The majority of respondents thought that it was important for physicians to be reevaluated every few years and that they need to do more to demonstrate competence. The authors noted that the competency of the individual physician seems to be overlooked in the current improvement efforts, perhaps because of the IOM (2001) report that emphasized improved systems over improved individuals within the system. A second reason is the limited number of reliable means available to measure physician quality. I believe that the example of my son's awful medical care and the subsequent bias in the evaluations of the reviewing cardiologists underscore this latter point. Later, I will propose a solution to this problem.

The Myth of Continuing Medical Education (CME)

Many states have requirements for continuing medical education of physicians; however, after talking to a number of doctors and looking at the specific CME requirements, I believe that in its current form, physician CME is a sham. It is a sham for 2 basic reasons. Firstly, even when a physician obtains CME as required by most state medical boards, there is no assurance that he takes that education in his specialty area, that it is relevant to his practice, that he mastered the content, or that the course content was sufficient to maintain competence. In an article published in 2005 in the *Journal of Continuing Education of Health Professionals (JCEHP)*, David Johnson and his coauthors state, "As currently structured and used by state medical boards, CME remains insufficient to ensure or verify continued competence [of physicians]." The nature of CME determines its effectiveness, as shown by a study published in *JAMA* (Davis et al., 1999) that concluded, "Our data show some evidence that interactive CME sessions that enhance participant activity and provide the opportunity to practice skills can effect change in professional practice and, on occasion, health care outcomes. Based on a small number of well-conducted trials, *didactic [lecture-based] sessions do not appear to be effective in changing physician performance.*" In another study that has direct bearing on my son's poor medical care, Davis and Taylor-Vaisey (1997), studying implementation of clinical practice guidelines (CPGs) between 1990 and 1996, reported, "The evidence shows serious deficiencies in the adoption of CPGs in practice. Future implementation strategies must overcome this failure through an understanding of the forces and variables influencing practice and through the use of methods that are practice- and community-based rather than didactic." A report in *JAMA* (Davis et al., 1995) concludes, "*Widely used CME delivery methods such as conferences have little direct impact on improving professional* practice. *More effective methods, such as systematic practice-based interventions and outreach visits, are seldom used by CME providers."*

Physicians have an increasing tendency to seek CME through online courses, but few studies have shown that these are effective. In one study, the conclusion seems to be mixed (Casebeer et al., 2004). The authors report that physicians having an average knowledge score of 58% before completing online courses between August 2002 and March 2003 had a knowledge score of 76% immediately after the courses, but 4 weeks later, that score dropped to 68%. Certainly, physicians must learn past their residency; however, 2 things are troubling. One is the fact that 4 weeks after the courses ended the average scores were in the range generally considered failing (68%), and one must wonder how much more decline would occur in the knowledge score as the months and years go on. Perhaps it would simply bottom out back at 58%.

Physicians are allowed to choose to do convenient or entertaining CME over relevant CME if they want to. There is no requirement to do CME in one's specialty. For example, one subject acceptable to the AMA for 24 hours of CME is called "Legal-Medical Issues" and can be taken in many exciting places aboard a cruise ship; try http://www.intcont.com/ to see where your physician might like to go! I like to sail; if I were a physician, I could take a number of courses aboard the catamaran called "Good Medicine," which sails out of the British Virgin Islands. I could earn 10 AMA category 1 CME credits by viewing a DVD on a computer each morning and taking an exam immediately afterward, all of which takes no more than 1-2 hours, leaving the remainder of each day for sailing. The proponents note that the cost might be tax deductible. I invite you to do a Web search using CME and cruise to observe the environments where CME can be obtained. I want to make it clear that combining a luxury cruise and CME does not necessarily make the CME of no value, but it seems very unlikely to produce a significant improvement in physician skills and knowledge.

The second reason that CME is ineffective in Texas is the way in which the TMB enforces the requirement that physicians complete CME each year. *According to the Executive Director of the TMB, in a letter to me dated January 16, 2006, only 1% of physician CME in Texas is verified each year.* There seems to be no sense at the TMB that during the time when a physician was not taking CME he may have been placing his patients at increased risk because of his ignorance. I think this cavalier attitude on the part of the TMB results from its recognition that physician CME in its current form has little effect on performance in clinical medicine, which is consistent with the articles I discussed above.

According to the AMA website http://www.ama-assn.org/ama/pub/category/2640.html (accessed 28 March 2006), Colorado, Connecticut, Montana, New York, and Oregon have no general requirements for physician CME. Some states and territories already require an average of 50 hours of CME each year; these are Guam, Illinois, Kansas, Maine, Massachusetts, Michigan, New Hampshire, New Jersey, North Carolina, Ohio, Pennsylvania, and Washington. No substantive CME in a physician's specialty is required except in Nevada, where 20 hours/year are required (and 4 hours of education about bioterrorism!). Some of the required CME courses are pain management/geriatric medicine (California), HIV/AIDS, domestic violence, child/dependent adult abuse (Iowa), infection control, child abuse (New York), HIV universal precautions/blood-borne pathogens (Rhode Island), ethics/professional responsibility (Texas), and end of life management (West Virginia). Of the 30 hours required by Virginia, at least 15 must be interactive training, and Massachusetts has a specific requirement to study board requirements and risk management. I assume this means board requirements in one's specialty. As I have indicated earlier, an understanding of risk management is essential to the competent practice of medicine and interactive CME produces better results than didactic teaching.

In conclusion, 4 things must occur before a Texan (or most Americans) can have a reasonable expectation that his cardiologist or other specialist knows what he is doing. Firstly, each CME course must have a content, delivery, and post-course test that ensure that the physician has learned and retained the material. Clearly this will require more than attendance at conferences, independent reading, online CME, or cruise-based CME. There must be interactive presentation of material and demonstrated retention of the material months after the course has ended. Secondly, CME must be performed in the supposed specialty of the physician and the course content must include all new CPGs in that specialty. Thirdly, *the amount of CME must be increased, at least in the life-critical specialties such as cardiology, to at least 40 hours per year for physicians who were not grandfathered into their specialty.* For specialists grandfathered into their specialty, CME must consist of at least 80 hours per year until the grandfathered specialist submits to and successfully reacquires board certification in his specialty. Finally, the TMB must ensure that every physician licensed in Texas has performed his CME each year. Physicians who have not must be placed on probation and this fact announced in the newspaper of the town where he practices. News of a physician's failure must also be entered into the medical board's public-access database on physicians. In addition to these changes in CME, *the law must not allow a physician to represent himself as a medical specialist if he lacks credentials from a recognized medical specialty board.*

Does Your Cardiologist Practice Preventive Care?

Most of us mistakenly assume that our physician will counsel us when we need to modify something within our control, undergo a simple screening test to rule out an insidious disease process, or protect ourselves from infectious disease threats. In an article entitled "Improving preventive care by prompting physicians" (Balas et al., 2000), the authors targeted 6 preventive medicine procedures: fecal occult blood test, mammogram, Pap smear, flu vaccine, pneumococcal vaccine, and tetanus vaccine. Published studies on the life-saving value of these preventive measures and the gap filled by prompting physicians to counsel their patients to have these tests or interventions performed led the authors to conclude that *more than 8,000 lives could be saved in the United States each year if physicians were prompted to counsel their patients when these common procedures need to be done.*

In a recent editorial in a medical journal (Wilson, 2006) the author asked, "Patient counseling and education: should doctors be doing more?" The editorial points out that only 3% of Americans adhere to all 4 key healthy lifestyle practices: no smoking, healthy weight, eating fruits and vegetables, and regular exercise. Since 1950 the percentage of overweight citizens has doubled to 65%, portending an epidemic of lifestyle-related diseases. Cardiovascular diseases will be foremost among those being "promoted" by our irresponsible lifestyles. The writer begins by noting that *even in the face of a compelling need to counsel patients about these factors, a large portion of physicians do not do this.* The barriers to doing it include the following: doctors may not be personally practicing a healthy lifestyle, doctors think they do not have time for disease-prevention counseling, doctors have not learned effective counseling techniques, and doctors often do not receive compensation for disease prevention counseling. I am no expert in counseling, but it is clear to me that a medical care system that places patients rather than physicians at its center will compel health professionals to effectively inform patients of the lifestyle changes they need to make and direct them to clinics for help.

Somehow *physicians, especially cardiologists, have been able to avoid accountability for their "duty to warn."* This concept is applied to product liability law. It requires the maker of a product to warn the user of dangers associated with its normal use and foreseeable misuses, and do this in a distinctly adequate manner. Furthermore, suggestions must be given for avoiding the anticipated danger. Why has the physician community been able to avoid this responsibility? Their product is your health and factors that endanger the value of that product should be identified and warned against.

In my opinion, preventive counseling in medical care is just as important as informed consent. Our culture is permeated with preventive warnings because we are a litigation-based society. When a cardiologist has a patient who is an obese smoker and never exercises, and the cardiologist fails to counsel the patient in writing on the lifestyle changes he needs to make, it is no different from a factory manager who fails to warn his workers of a dangerous product in use, or a pilot who fails to warn his passengers when he knows that his airplane is entering a zone of extreme turbulence. If someone dies or is injured because they were not warned, then someone is held legally responsible. Simply put, *it is negligent and unethical not to explicitly counsel a patient who needs a lifestyle change to manage his risk of heart disease or other illness. That advice must be put in writing.*

Cardiac Examination Skills by Non-cardiologists

An informed and trained physician can determine much about the health of his patient's heart during a cardiac examination; however, the ability to perform a cardiac examination seems to be on the decline (Vukanovic-Criley et al., 2006). The barriers identified by the authors to effective cardiac examination training include lack of appropriate patient examples, lack of bedside time, *promotion of more expensive diagnostic testing*, and lack of knowledgeable instructors. The authors used a validated 50-question test to assess the cardiac examination skills of 860 participants ranging from medical students to cardiac fellows. The mean competency score for all participants was only 59%. The "good news" is that the 85 cardiology fellows scored on average about 72%. The authors postulated that the physicians' failure to integrate visual and auditory information during the cardiac examination may contribute to the overall poor performance. The authors concluded that *"cardiac examination skills do not improve after the 3rd year of medical school and may decline after years of practice, which has important implications for medical decision making, patient safety, cost-effective care, and CME."* I have had first-hand experience with this inability to perform a quality cardiac examination and the resultant excess patient costs (see "Laura's Story" in Chapter 3).

The skill of primary care clinicians in identifying patients at risk for an acute myocardial infarction is critical. In a study of 966 patients admitted to hospitals with a myocardial infarction and no history of coronary heart disease, it was reported that 27% of these patients had primary care visits during the preceding month in which symptoms of coronary artery disease were reported (Sequist et al., 2006). Of this group, two fifths (106/261) were not referred for hospital care. The authors note that this high rate of "missed opportunities" may be due to lack of structured evaluation of patients and lack of procedures for triage. For example, only half of the patients received an ECG before leaving the primary physician's office. An ECG can indicate when a patient with symptoms referable to coronary artery disease needs further medical attention.

The answer to the question posed by the chapter title is troubling. If your cardiologist is not board certified in cardiology, then no one says your cardiologist knows what he is doing. If he is board certified, it is physicians on medical boards who say that your cardiologist knows what he is doing. But actually all they can say is that at one time your grandfathered cardiologist passed an examination and was deemed a cardiologist for life. He may have learned little cardiology since then. I asked a catheterization technician why the older cardiologist who did the left heart catheterization on Alex was still using 7F catheters in 2002 when the medical literature seemed to say that the standard was to use smaller 5F and 4F catheters. His answer to me was, "I guess that's the way he learned it." If a non-grandfathered cardiologist maintains competency by fulfilling medical board requirements, and that is a big if, then every 10 years the ABIM can attest that he has practiced cardiology, has not been caught doing anything terribly wrong, and has managed to stuff enough information in his head to pass another examination. You might ask how often you would fly if commercial pilots were held to the same standards.

Chapter 9
Lessons from Other Professions: Pilots and Auto Mechanics

It's Not Easy to Be a Doctor

Two facets of being a physician in a life-critical specialty distinguish it and make it a difficult occupation. *The first is that the lives of patients depend on the ability of the physician to diagnose and treat the illness. Holding the life of another human being in your hands is a humbling responsibility (or at least it ought to be). The second is that the correct approaches to diagnosis and treatment are constantly changing.* Are there other professions that experience the same sort of responsibility and change? I think commercial airline pilots experience the responsibility because they hold the lives of hundreds of people in their hands each time they fly a packed commercial jet. But the piloting of a jet does not change much over the years, so pilots are not subjected to the continuous changes that occur in medicine. After some consideration, I decided that the rate of change of professional skills needed should be comparable for physicians and master automobile mechanics. Servicing automobiles that are constantly changing due to competition is not unlike diagnosing and treating patients with constantly changing illnesses, using new tools and guidelines. How do pilots and master mechanics maintain their skills, and can we apply their models to the physician in a life-critical specialty?

Pilots and Physicians

From a customer's point of view, the importance of a pilot's skill and knowledge and that of a physician in a life-critical specialty are similar. Most rational people would not board a commercial jet aircraft if they thought the pilot had been certified as a pilot on a DC3 many years ago and had never trained on a modern type of aircraft since his initial training. Furthermore, we would never suppose that the good will of the pilot, and his fear of dying with us, would be sufficient to cause him to remain cognizant of emergency procedures and maneuvers, changing flight operations, and upgrades to the aircraft that he routinely flies. We would not do this because we would not want to risk our life aboard an aircraft piloted by a person who has unpracticed piloting skills and outdated knowledge. Periodically, we are made painfully aware of the danger of flying when an airplane crash kills several hundred people at one time. Most often the cause of the crash is *not* pilot error because stringent piloting requirements are rigorously dictated by federal laws and strictly enforced.

In the same way as we entrust pilots with our lives every time we fly, we also entrust physicians with our lives when they diagnose and treat us for a serious illness or give us guidance on how to prevent a serious illness. Yet we have somehow been satisfied to allow physicians to self-regulate their profession, setting standards for continuing education that are generally ineffective as far as maintaining skills and knowledge in medical specialties is concerned. I think there are 3 reasons for this. First, physicians routinely get away with the practice of unskilled and uninformed medicine because their victims do not even know that they have been harmed by it, and because there is no place for a harmed patient to register a complaint short of a lawsuit.

Secondly, uninformed and inattentive medical practice kills patients one at a time in diverse locations, so there are no evening news bulletins to focus everyone's attention on the fact that today in America about 800 people—babies, frightened children, loving mothers, proud fathers, doting grandmas, and story-telling grandpas—died because of medical errors. In my hometown of Houston there is a news commentator named Marvin Zindler who, each evening on the news, lists the names and nature of the violations committed by restaurants that have been inspected by the health department. Suppose there was a commentator who each day reported the physicians who had not completed their *relevant* CME or had been found otherwise negligent in their practice. Suppose there was a commentator who listed hospitals found deficient during inspections and described what those deficiencies were. Suppose we actually knew and announced exactly who had died or been injured because of medical errors and who committed those errors. How quickly the system would become patient-centered!

Thirdly, *medical professionals have a strong tendency not to report mistakes*. A recent press release from the Harvard School of Public Health (2006) makes reference to an article entitled "Problem doctors: Is there a system level solution?" published in the *Annals of Internal Medicine* (Leape and Fromson et al., 2006). The news release asserts, "Doctors have not done it [reported problem physicians] because they have not wanted to be critical of colleagues, and there was no mechanism short of curtailing practice or taking a doctor's license away. *But everyone knows at least one doctor with a problem: it's the elephant in the room*" (bold type mine). Realistically, we patients, or potential patients, must recognize that human nature makes us all reluctant to "snitch" on our colleagues regardless of our profession. *We must create a physician monitoring system in which those outside the profession initiate actions against bad doctors without having to sue them*, and we must devise a plan of CME, akin to recurrent training for pilots, that rigorously forces specialists to remain knowledgeable and skillful in their specialty. Ultimately, we cannot rely on physicians to report their uninformed, belligerent, unethical, and dangerous colleagues to a regulatory body; it just is not going to happen.

Recurrent Training of Pilots

Pilots and flight engineers of commercial passenger aircraft (Group II aircraft) are required by the Federal Aviation Administration (FAA) to complete 25 hours of training 2 times a year to maintain their license to fly. That training for pilots must include the following: (1) flight training in an approved simulator in maneuvers and procedures set forth in the certificate holder's approved low-altitude wind-shear flight training program and (2) flight training in maneuvers and procedures set forth in appendix F to this part of the rules, or in a flight training program approved by the FAA administrator. This is a convoluted way of saying what pilots must learn or relearn each year.

A commercial pilot has told me that these rules basically amount to this: Several hours of training, twice per year are required in full motion simulators. The training is specific to the type of aircraft flown by the pilot, and performance testing is preceded by an oral examination. A typical test lasts 7 hours. The instructor can train the pilot to some extent, but the pilot must pass the simulator test in no more than 2 tries. If the pilot in recurrent training fails the test a second time, he is subject to losing his license. In addition, 8 hours of basic indoctrination is required each year to review company policies, FAA regulations, and changes in procedures. Another 8 hours of training is required each year in "resource management," which focuses on interactions between the captain and crew. The goal is to ensure that each flight crew functions as a team regardless of which individual is filling each role. A ground school of 8 hours is also required to review aircraft systems and basically reiterate what can be broken on a specific type of plane without preventing it from being flown safely. The trainee must pass a test at the end of this recurrent training. A 1-hour computer-based course in winter operations is also required each year.

By my count about 40 to 50 hours of recurrent annual training is required of commercial pilots. Much of this training is "hands on" in simulators and is specific to the aircraft that the pilot flies. This is necessary because the lives of people depend on pilots knowing what they are doing and because passengers have little control in selecting the quality of pilots who fly their aircraft. This is in stark contrast to the haphazard requirements for physician CME, which I summarized earlier.

If they are lucky, patients have some time and can select a physician based on hearsay; however, in a case like my son's we had no effective choice in which cardiologists saw him or which physician wrote his hospital summary. Many elder Americans enjoy traveling in this country. How are they supposed to identify a competent cardiologist in an unfamiliar place if they need one? The physician's situation is precisely like the situation with pilots: our lives depend on the ability of the physician or pilot, and we have no effective means to select ones with demonstrated competency. *Legislation is necessary to ensure that all physicians in life-critical specialties are trained annually in their specialty, just as pilots are retrained annually.*

Master Mechanics and Doctors

We have all been frustrated at one time or another by difficulty in getting our cars repaired effectively and quickly. Cars change rapidly in both technology and design, so the modern mechanic must not only learn to repair cars, he must be constantly learning to service new models. When I was a kid, there were fewer than 10 choices of cars (all American) to purchase and models did not change much from year to year, but now each manufacturer has 5-15 models of its own, so that there are hundreds of models to choose from and these models change from year to year. Mechanics must be smart and willing to perform meaningful continuing education if they hope to do their job well. When they do not do a good job of diagnosing and repairing a vehicle problem, the customer will generally know that the job was botched soon after he drives away from the dealer. If the mechanic does not want angry customers returning often to his shop, then he must do the job right the first time. This is not the case with physicians. They can and frequently do make mistakes that their patients are never aware of, but they are not held accountable in the same way as an auto mechanic is. In fact, it is not uncommon for physicians to receive payment for correcting their secret mistakes.

If you are a master diagnostic technician working for Toyota, you have already spent a great deal of your time and money achieving that status, but then you are required to take one 8-hour course for each new model introduced. About 4 new models are introduced each year, so this alone requires about 32 hours per year of continuing *specific* education. In addition to this, you must attend an annual 8-hour in-class technical conference. Each year, in the shop where you work, you must pass the master diagnostic technician test, which involves practical application of knowledge. You must prepare for this test on your own time and that typically takes about 12 hours. If you do not pass the test with a grade of 80% or better, you lose the status and pay that come with the master diagnostic technician designation. ***Thus to remain a top mechanic for Toyota you must acquire about 50 hours of specific continuing education each year and you get tested over what you have learned!***

The 17-Year Gap

Please compare the preparedness a top mechanic has in diagnosing a problem with your car to that of a medical specialist's average preparedness to diagnose and treat your health problem. Research has shown that on average about 15-17 years is required from the time clinically-relevant knowledge from a randomized controlled trial is published until it is adopted at the clinical level by 50% of physicians (Balas and Boren, 2000). Suppose you had a 5-year-old Camry and took it to the dealer complaining that the steering had suddenly become erratic and the car was dangerous. How would you feel if the repair service told you that the steering was a new design the year your car was built, so you had to wait 12 more years to bring your car in because it takes 17 years from the time a new model is manufactured until half their best mechanics have assimilated the knowledge to repair the model you drive? You would never stand for this because you have choices in which car to buy and which dealer does the repairs. Sadly, in the current medical care system you are often not going to get the latest diagnosis and treatment options because there is no meaningful competition based on quality of care. In the area of southeast Houston where I live, people have anecdotal information on which hospitals and physicians to stay away from, but what happens if you are taken by ambulance to one of the "dangerous" hospitals? What happens if you are in an unfamiliar city as my son was, and you do not know if you are being taken to a competent hospital?

Chapter 10
Targets for Change: Patient Safety Legislation

Where Do We Begin?

I am reluctant to start this section by telling you what changes are needed that I will *not* be concerned with, but I will do that anyway. The present American medical system is a wreck. That wreck consists of at least the following failures: it is too costly and is becoming a serious economic burden to our society; the delivery is fragmented among many providers; it is not equitably administered to all Americans; it has failed to improve American life expectancy above that of many less-developed countries; physicians are frustrated by being second-guessed by insurance companies that are too slow to pay claims; scientific medical information is ever increasing, yet the average time to integrate it into clinical practice (to 50% implementation) is 17 years; physicians have little accountability for their many errors; at least 300,000 Americans die each year from medical errors; and patients are isolated from their care by secrecy and doctoring of their records. Here I am not going to deal with the problems of excessive cost, fragmentation, unequal access, and physician frustrations. *The targets for change I will focus on are these: 1) ensuring that physicians know what they are doing and 2) transforming the present non-system of care into a transparent system centered on patients and their needs.*

A transparent, patient-centered medical care system with technically competent specialists can be created independently of how other problems with the current system are solved. For example, Bartlett and Steele (2006), in their book *Critical Condition*, have proposed that the federal government take over the current costly, fragmented, and inequitable system. I share their deep concerns with the current system, but I am reluctant to hand over the whole mess to the federal government. You saw how the DHHS was incapable of dealing with my simple question of whether my son's medical records had been tampered with after his death. Nonetheless, it may be time to consider a federal solution. Regardless of who administers the transformed system, it must be patient-centered and have medical specialists who know what they are doing. Thus, I will deal only with these last 2 facets of a new health care system (patient-centeredness and physician knowledge), and leave the other deficiencies of the current system for others to bend, weld, or hammer into place.

In the sections below I will use the experience with my son's cardiologists and more objective information in a book from the IOM that was published in 2001. This one is called *Crossing the Quality Chasm: A New Health System for the 21ˢᵗ Century*. It lays out an agenda for radical reform of the medical care system in the U.S.

A Patient-centered Medical System

Your Medical Records

Laws must be written to require physicians to offer medical records to their patients after every office visit and hospital stay. The authors of an article in the *Archives of Internal Medicine* on adoption of patient-centered medical care practices report that of more than 1800 experienced primary-care physicians who were surveyed, 83% were in favor of sharing medical records with their patients (apparently 17% were not) (Audet et al., 2006). Seventy-four percent of the doctors experienced problems with the availability of patients' medical records or test results at the time of a scheduled visit. If patients had their medical records and test data themselves, they could ensure its availability at a scheduled office visit and be prepared to ask informed questions. We patients must be allowed to become full participants in our medical care; we cannot leave access to medical records to the discretion of practicing physicians!

Furthermore, the law must require that these records be written in a way that an informed layperson can understand. It is absurd that medical records are still handwritten by some specialists (Exhibit 13). When I asked for a copy that I could read, I was told by an assistant to the doctor that they *never* type their records. After I made 2 inquiries, a nurse in the urologist's office interpreted the writing for me. Clearly written records must be available to the patient within 5 working days of the visit or hospital stay. Patients could have the option of declining to receive the records and could sign a form to that effect, but the physician or one of his staff must take the initiative to provide the records. The physician could charge a nominal fee for this service. If a patient is in a hospital for an extended stay, then any records more than 5 days old must be offered by the hospital staff to the patient or his designated representative. *A patient with a copy of his medical records can become an informed patient capable of participating in his own care*; this is nearly impossible without the records. Furthermore, this law will inhibit physicians from doctoring the records later to protect themselves from accountability for their errors.

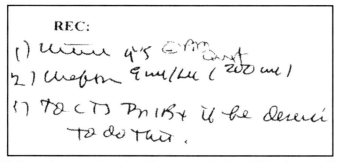

Exhibit 13. Part of a report I received from an urologist in 2006 after an office visit.

An interesting editorial was recently published by a physician who at age 52 became a patient when he was diagnosed with a rare disease (peripheral neuropathy from primary amyloidosis) (Neubauer, 2006). The doctor-now-patient lamented the absurdity of "privacy paranoia" caused by the Health Insurance Portability and Accountability Act. One of the results of this act is the physician's reduced ability to interact with patients. For example, email communications between physicians and patients are much constrained. The author concluded that such rules "are a throwback to times when illness was cloaked in secrecy." From my perspective it is ridiculous to see such silly constraints in the interest of privacy and virtually no legal control of the quality of medical care. I suspect that physicians have some interest in keeping secrecy. For example, I talked by phone to the director of Hospital 1, where Alex was primarily treated, and complained that the older cardiologist had passed false information to his colleagues about Alex being offered a pacemaker, and they had written it into Alex's medical records from that hospital. He said an internal hospital investigation of Alex's care would be conducted. I asked him to ensure that the investigation team in his hospital be given records from Hospital 2 showing that Alex was offered a loop monitor and *not* a pacemaker. The director told me that they could not look at or consider records from another hospital as part of their investigation. Privacy, you know! The director did tell me that he remembered that a *rumor* was going around after Alex died that he was offered a pacemaker.

The IOM book lists what a patient should expect from his health care system. I quote the vision from page 63 of that book: "You can know what you wish to know, when you wish to know it. Your medical record is yours to keep, to read, and to understand. The rule is: 'Nothing about you without you.'" This has particular relevance to my son's death. If he and I had had rapid access to his ECGs showing that his QTc dropped from 479 ms to 390 ms overnight, we would have noted the dramatic change in his QTc and asked his cardiologists about that change since they had expressed concern about the higher number. Apparently, they never saw this change. We could have been an active part of his care rather than passively receiving information from cardiologists who, as it turned out, were too uninformed and hurried to look at the medical data. Furthermore, if we had had access to his medical record, the lie about him and his parents refusing a pacemaker and an electroencephalogram would not have been allowed.

Therefore, the law will further specify that the medical record cannot contain a statement about the patient's refusal of any treatment unless the treatment has been recommended and explained in writing and the patient has signed a form acknowledging that the treatment has been recommended in writing. If the patient refuses the recommendation in writing, then, and only then, the physician can enter this fact into the patient's medical record. Patients will be encouraged to report deviations from this law to the transformed TMB (see below).

Implementation of this law will require a major change in the mindset of physicians and hospital administrators, so it will need to be phased in over 1 year. During the first year the TMB will set up a patient-reporting database and use it to accumulate data on physicians and hospitals as patients send in complaints about limited access to their records. At the end of the one year grace period, the database will be purged of all complaints against physicians and hospitals, and they will have a fresh start. Once the phase-in period is over, enforcement should be by the TMB using a database format. Prospective patients of a given physician or hospital could visit this database and see how often patients have complained about the physician or hospital not freely providing medical records as specified in the law. Physicians and hospitals that violate this law persistently after the 2nd year will be identified by the TMB and placed on probation. *The TMB will be required by law to announce that probation in newspapers of the city where the hospital is located or the physician practices medicine.*

A second phase of this law, perhaps implemented after the second year, would require that a patient be able to place his own comments into his medical record, which must, by then, be in an electronic format. The patient should never be able to change the physician's portion of the medical record. However, for example, I would have entered into my son's medical records that I offered to get his Air Force ECG, but the older cardiologist was not interested. I would have entered our concern about his need for a neurological evaluation as a possible cause of his syncope and the family doctor's explanation that Alex's syncope was not neurological. I would have entered into the record that I voiced concern about his hypokalemia and was told that it was being addressed (nurse) or not of concern (older cardiologist). Selected entries could be "negotiated" and signed by patient and physician. ***Imagine the empowerment when you can place your questions and their answers in your medical record!***

Falsification of *Your* Medical Records

As I have shown you, the weight of evidence is that my son's older cardiologist and the PIT conspired to modify my son's medical records to show that an electroencephalogram was recommended and refused by my son and that a pacemaker was also recommended and refused. The older cardiologist spread the pacemaker lie to his colleagues and placed a direct falsification in the "DEATH SUMMARY" when he stated that my son's cardiac MRI was negative (Exhibit 14A); in fact it was aborted or "cancelled undiagnostic" (Exhibit 14 B). The older cardiologist's statement in Exhibit 14A about the family requesting an autopsy is false. I agreed with the older cardiologist's declaration to me that *he* intended to obtain an autopsy of my son's heart and brain. I remember this clearly because we were told that we would have to pay for an autopsy if we requested one. I leave you to ponder why the older cardiologist "forgot" to mention that he had done a left heart catheterization on Alex, and also why the Dallas pathologist was not informed of this before he looked for injury to my son's heart.

Placing or enabling your medical colleagues to place false statements in medical records cannot be tolerated. In a case like my son's, this is tantamount to tampering with evidence. ***Legislation must clearly communicate to physicians that they are criminally liable if they are caught "doctoring" medical records in a case where those records could become evidence in a legal action.*** The legislation must include an enforcement plan. Providing medical records to patients soon after an office visit or hospital stay will alleviate some of the pressure on physicians because the patient will have been provided with his record, and if he does not complain about an apparent error in the record, then the physician can assert that the patient knew of the error and did nothing to correct it.

```
A
NAME: JAMES, ALEX          MR#  000535093
PHYSICIAN: <DELETED>       LOCATION:  MIC5515-1
ADMISSION DATE: 09/15/02   DISCHARGE DATE: 09/18/02

DEATH SUMMARY:

This is an unfortunate 19-year old college student who had an out-of-hospital cardiac
arrest on September 15, while jogging. It is unclear how long he was down but ACLS
protocol was instituted on site and he had multiple shocks for ventricular fibrillation and
prolonged CPR on the scene. Sinus rhythm was eventually restored and he was admitted
to the medical ICU at [Hospital 1]. He had had a past history of extensive workup for
syncope. **At that time he had a negative treadmill test, negative echocardiogram,
negative MRI and negative electrophysiologic study.**
...
He continued to deteriorate and eventually became asystolic on the evening of 9/17. He
was pronounced dead at approximately 10:30 p.m.

CAUSE OF DEATH: SEVERE CARDIOGENIC SHOCK SECONDARY TO OUT-OF-
HOSPITAL CARDIAC ARREST.

The patient's family requested a limited autopsy to the heart and brain and arrangements
were made for this to be performed.
-------------------------------------------------------------------------------------------------
B
Exam Date: 08/21/2002   Arrival Time: 1257   Status:   CANCELLED
Entered By:        MRI-MDP- <deleted> 08/21/2002  1257
**CANCELLED**UNDIAGNOSTIC** By: MRI-LMC  08/23/2002 1242
```

Exhibit 14. The older cardiologist's entry in Alex's medical record, called his "death summary" (A), and the MRI record sent to me by Hospital 1 (B).
Compare the older cardiologist's statement about Alex's cardiac MRI (A) and the hospital's record of the MRI (B). He also omitted any mention of Alex's left heart catheterization, which he had done himself. Also missing is any mention of Alex's highly abnormal ECGs (Exhibit 9, page 44).

Informed Consent Must Be Genuine

At present I can find no specific law that requires physicians to receive informed consent from a patient before performing an invasive procedure that may put the patient's life at risk. According to the Director of the TMB, in a letter to me dated January 16, 2006, failing to give informed consent falls under a general law designed to protect patients from physicians who "fail to practice medicine in an acceptable professional manner consistent with public health and welfare," which is statute 164.051 (a) (6). The Director refused to examine his records in response to my question about how often this sort of physician failure was due to lack of informed consent.

This non-specific approach by the TMB is not sufficient to ensure that each patient receives authentic informed consent before going under the knife. *The state of Texas must legally define what constitutes informed consent and then enforce its application to every patient in Texas.*

The IOM has declared in their summary of what a patient should expect from a health care system, "You [the patient] will be known and respected as an individual. Your choices and preferences will be sought and honored...When your needs are special, the care system will adapt to meet you on your own terms." The AMA posted their definition of informed consent on their website in September, 1998—4 years before my son was deceived into giving his "informed consent" for left heart catheterization (http://www.ama-assn.org/ama/pub/category/4608.html). The elements of their definition can be summarized as follows:

1) The physician planning to do the invasive procedure should do the disclosure and discussing.
2) The patient should be told his diagnosis.
3) The physician should disclose the nature and purpose of the invasive procedure.
4) The physician should disclose the risks and benefits of the invasive procedure.
5) The physician should present alternatives to the invasive procedure with their risks and benefits.
6) The physician should present the risks and benefits of not receiving the invasive procedure.

Strangely, the AMA website goes on to assert that not only medical ethics but legal requirements in all 50 states require informed consent. This does not seem to be the case in Texas. The hospital where my son was cajoled into signing informed consent forms failed on the AMA's elements 1, 5, and 6. The cardiologist was not present when informed consent was elicited from Alex (although he had given him the Pete Maravich scare speech earlier), he was not told about any alternatives (and there were several), and the risks and benefits of not receiving the planned catheterization were not discussed. Element 2 was irrelevant since there was no diagnosis (but there should have been), element 3 was reasonably well addressed, and element 4 was discussed in an uninformative way since no one present knew the probability of any of the bad outcomes. The AMA site has a long paragraph on how the physician (and his attorney) ought to minimize his risk of litigation associated with informed consent. The AMA (2001) has summarized the physician-patient relationship this way in the

9th point of their version of the Hippocratic Oath: "A physician shall, while caring for a patient, regard responsibility to the patient as paramount." If only it were so!

Informed consent forms should also provide an estimate to the patient of the cost of the proposed procedure. Patients cannot expect their physicians to be unbiased when advice in one direction will earn them many thousands of dollars, and a choice to not have the procedure will earn them nothing. Informed consent must include all reasonably anticipated hospital and physician fees associated with the procedure if it goes as expected. Medical costs are increasingly being shifted to the individual and many people will not spend tens of thousands of dollars on a medical procedure unless they are thoroughly convinced that it has significant value to them or their loved one.

Informed consent between a patient and physician for an invasive procedure must be legally defined to include written descriptions of all reasonable alternatives to the proposed procedure (including doing nothing), the rationale for the invasive procedure, the quantitative risk of adverse outcomes when that risk is known, and the expected monetary costs of the procedure and alternatives; the physician administering the invasive test will sign the form as will the patient.

Enforcement of informed consent laws must gain specificity and teeth. In a column dated January 20, 2005, in the *Houston Chronicle*, Rick Casey stated, "Under Texas law a person must have effective consent to cut on another person. It is not effective consent according to the penal code, if it is induced by force, threat, or fraud." He states further, "Aggravated assault is intentionally, knowingly, or recklessly causing serious bodily injury to another." Alex's cardiologists *intentionally* cut on his body, *knowing* that he could be injured or even die from their invasion of his body, they elicited his permission to do this by the *threat* that he needed them to cut on him to rule out life-threatening illness, and they committed *fraud* (deceit perpetrated for profit) because they did not inform him of his alternative choices to invasion of his body. I found that the current law in Texas is not as effective as Mr. Casey suggests. Twice I went in a circular loop with the city Police Department, the County Prosecutor's Office, and the Texas State Attorney General's Office trying to identify a law-enforcement agency that would investigate my claim that my son was not given informed consent. None of them would take my deposition. Each informed me that it was not their job to enforce such laws. I could find no agency in Texas that cared to get involved in enforcement of failure to give informed consent to my son. *Suspected violations of the informed consent law will receive criminal investigation. It seems to me that the county prosecutor's office of the county where the alleged offense occurred should be specifically given the task and funding to investigate claims of physicians failing to give informed consent.* How many times do you suppose physicians would have to be investigated for failure to give informed consent before they would all comply with this most important law?

Transforming the Texas (and other State) Medical Board

Patient Advocacy

In Texas the governor appoints the president of the TMB. At present this individual is a physician and lawyer. Currently the president appoints persons to the TMB and the ratio of 12 physicians to 7 public members is specified by statute [Sec 152.003 of the Medical Practice Act]. In my opinion, this must be reversed so that more technically-oriented, non-physicians are on the board than physicians. As I noted earlier, there is a natural tension between patient complainants and the physician community. *The TMB's stacking of the deck heavily in favor of the physicians has a chilling effect on patients' rights regarding complaints against their health care providers.*

A Farewell to Secrecy

The medical profession has been protected from accountability far too long because of the secret processes used to determine the culpability of practitioners. To my knowledge, no other profession enjoys such secret deliberations. For example, as I write this section a major controversy is being debated *in public* over the publication in *Science* magazine of an article on the cloning of human embryos from which stem cells were extracted. The journal editors had gone through the usual process of anonymous reviews by 2-3 experts in the field and the article was published in May 2005, but it now seems that major parts of the data may have been fabricated. No one is claiming that the scientist in question, Hwang Woo-suk of the Seoul National University, deserves secrecy until the final conclusion is determined. The "holy grail" in science is scientific truth and the personal reputation of an individual scientist is secondary. *I would argue that currently the "holy grail" in medical care is the protection of all physicians, even those who are uninformed, reckless, and unethical, from accountability for their mistakes.* Secondary to this is the protection of medical institutes from accountability. I note that any information developed during an investigation by the Joint Commission on Accreditation of Healthcare Organizations (JCAHO) on medical errors made in a specific institution cannot be publicly disclosed. Somewhere, a distant priority is the protection of patients from medical errors that kill hundreds of thousands of patients each year. This situation must be turned on its head. *When a patient dies or is seriously injured under circumstances remotely suggestive of uninformed medical care, the TMB must conduct its investigation in an open fashion.*

The IOM (2001) has clearly asserted in its rule #7 that secrecy must become a thing of the past. Quoting from their patient expectations, "Your care will be confidential, but the care system will not keep secrets from you. You can know whatever you wish to know about the care that affects you and your loved ones." In another place they further characterize their rule #7: "The pursuit of confidentiality is not a reason for hiding the system's performance failures from those who depend on the system. This new rule calls for health systems to be accountable to the public; to do their work openly; to make their results known to the public and professionals alike; and to build trust through disclosure, even of the systems' own problems." *Laws must be changed to transform the TMB from a den of secret-keepers to a trusted agency of the State of Texas known for openly, fairly, and passionately accomplishing its goal of patient safety in the health care system.*

The TMB will assert that losing the secrecy of the process will put a chilling effect on physicians coming forward with information and the board's experts being honest. These concerns can be addressed by simple statute. Any physician who does not cooperate with a TMB investigation is to be placed on publicly-announced probation. If that fails to elicit cooperation, then the physician's license to practice in Texas is temporarily suspended. The names of experts should be withheld; however, their opinions must be available for open review. Without this openness, there is no hope of quality control on the physicians who render their opinions. I also think they should be paid much more than $100 per hour for their work and there should be a requirement that each specialist practicing in Texas may be expected to give up to 8 hours of paid service to the TMB each year.

What would quality control of the TMB and the DPRC expert evaluation process look like? The complainant's written questions (not just a pile of medical records, as now practiced) must be openly available and provided directly to the expert, and the expert must answer each of the complainant's questions according to his knowledge of applicable standards to the medical situation and according to the practice of evidence-based medicine. *An expert opinion unsubstantiated by citing of the applicable clinical guidelines and standards will not be accepted by the DPRC.* The IOM firmly supports this approach to the practice of medicine. Their rule

#5 asserts, "You [the patient] will have care based on the best available scientific knowledge. The system promises you excellence as its standard. Your care will not vary illogically from doctor to doctor or from place to place. The system will promise you all the care that can help you, and will help you avoid care that cannot help you." This promise requires that all physicians know what they are doing and that complainants' issues be addressed from an evidence-based perspective.

Transforming Medical Education

One of the key targets for change is the way residents are selected and trained. To quote a recent editorial in *JAMA* (Leach and Philibert, 2006), "Residents who experience an adverse event were equally likely to implicate inadequate supervision (20%) and excessive duty hours (19%) as possible causes, followed by problems with patient handoffs." These observations resonate in my mind as I think about the careless medical care provided to Alex. The PIT was apparently under the supervision of a "real" doctor at the time she wrote my son's hospital discharge report and also at the time she saw him for an office visit a few days later. I think a skilled physician could look at either of her records and tell that she was doing a marginal job. Her skill should have been questioned, but apparently it was not. While the "patient handoff issue" in the quotation above refers to the imparting of information from the staff on one shift to the staff on the next shift, this same issue at a different level applies to Alex's care. Why was the responsibility for Alex's hospital discharge summary handed off to the PIT, a non-cardiologist, who was training in a different specialty? Why was the responsibility for his follow-up visit handed off to her? The *JAMA* editorial ends by stating that high-quality physician learning and high-quality patient care are impossible without each other. Attention to both is needed. I heartily agree.

Continuing medical education for physicians cannot continue in its current form because medical knowledge is growing at an unprecedented rate and too many Americans are dying from uninformed medical care. For example, the average number of registered clinical trials in cardiology increased from 15 per year in the late 1960s to more than 900 per year in the early 1990s (Cochrane Control Trials Register, cited in Balas and Boren, 2000). Most of these studies do not produce data that require a change in clinical practices; however, somehow the important studies must be identified and this knowledge packaged and transferred to practicing cardiologists. This is a huge burden of new knowledge each year and cardiologists must acknowledge that they cannot maintain competency without plenty of help. For physicians in life-critical specialties such as cardiovascular disease, the CME requirement must be that each physician annually demonstrates competence in his or her knowledge of that specialty. *Competence includes a working knowledge of the latest medical guidelines, knowledge of the latest scientific developments on proper uses of drugs, knowledge of patient safety laws, and knowledge of new diagnostic and treatment methods that have proven effective.*

I can envision a 40-hour course given each year in medical specialties that encompasses these requirements. The course concludes with a comprehensive examination that must be passed for the physician to continue to represent himself as a specialist to his patients. Remember, we are transforming to a patient-centered health care system, and patients have the right to informed and evidence-based medical care. I believe this is consistent with selected recommendations of the Conjoint Committee on CME (Spivey, 2005). The committee's recommendation 3 was that each specialty and subspecialty should develop core curricula and that the knowledge, skills, and attitudes should be in terms of [clinical] competencies. According to the committee's recommendation 4, the CME should contain valid content defined as emerging, evidence-based medicine free of bias on the part of those involved as teachers and learners in the process.

By requiring this approach to CME, we will be able to short-circuit the 17-year knowledge lag down to only a year or 2. Balas and Boren (2000), citing a collection of studies, showed that the time from the entry into bibliographic medical databases of a paper reporting clinically-relevant research findings to the appearance of these findings in a review paper or textbook was 6 to 13 years, and the time from publication of a review paper or textbook to implementation of the findings was 9 more years. *If CME goes directly from the published study to placing the finding before those who can implement the change in a clinical setting, the clinician can offer his patient the latest medical care advances.* Specialists are going to have to take the time to identify critical new findings. This may be naïve, but I can envision a system in which all cardiologists identify 10 critical new studies each year and report their opinions into a nationwide database. Experts would compile the "votes" and prepare an interactive 40-hour course that summarizes the clinical application of the most-identified studies. Your eligibility to take the course depends on your submission of 10 entries. If a cardiologist does not submit candidate studies, then he cannot take the course, and then he cannot keep his certification of competency as a cardiologist.

The IOM's perspective on this is as follows: "The health care system today is too tolerant of mismatches between knowledge and action; that is it is too accepting of both omission and waste. As a result, care is too often unreliable, advice and answers are inconsistent, and clinical practice varies without well founded rationale." In the new system every patient will have care based on the best available scientific knowledge, and this will not happen unless physicians continue to learn. The law will mandate the role of the TMB in CME. It will ensure that 100% of all physicians in Texas have performed meaningful CME each year. The current 1% CME verification is a joke. The new system will require a TMB-administered computer database to which each physician submits evidence of having done his CME. From this it will be simple to identify doctors who have not complied with the CME law.

One of the most startling discoveries I made as I prepared to write this book was that cardiologists who were board-certified before 1990 by the American Board of Internal Medicine (ABIM) are not required to demonstrate that they are maintaining their ability to practice informed cardiology. Because state-mandated CME does not specify that the CME be done in a physician's specialty, and there is little enforcement of CME anyway, a cardiologist can practice for decades without learning anything new in cardiology except what he derives from seeing patients and interacting with colleagues. This situation cannot continue because it places too many cardiology patients at risk, and some will die as a result. Since the key to my son's diagnosis and treatment was in his ECGs, and none of his cardiologists saw it, a quote from a recent article by 2 physicians seems apropos. "In recent years, important new information resulted from careful analysis of the ECG in patients with ischemic and non-ischemic heart disease. The trend toward increasing specialization in cardiology threatens the implementation of this new ECG knowledge in the daily practice of the cardiologist. *It remains essential, therefore, to stress that both old and new ECG knowledge should be in the core curriculum of every cardiologist, not only during his or her training, but especially also during postgraduate education"(Wellens and Gorgels, 2004).* I wish I could paste this sign on the dashboard of every cardiologist's Mercedes, Porsche, or Lexus to remind them of their responsibility.

I believe the solution to this is to mandate by law that physicians in critical specialties who are grandfathered by the board in that specialty must complete 80 hours per year of specialty-specific CME and 20 additional hours of general CME. The specialty-specific CME must include examinations verifying that the material has been learned and *retained* by the physician. Assessment of retention would require a follow up examination several months after the course has been completed. This should be a no-nonsense process. If the specialist flunks the retention examination, then he is placed on probation and that fact is announced in his hometown newspaper and on the TMB website. Remember, we are placing the patient's right to informed medical care above the physician's rights as a care provider to practice medicine in the state of Texas.

An alternative for these grandfathered specialists is that they can retake board examinations in their specialty and remain subject to the newer rules of the board that governs the process of maintenance of competency. This would place them on an equal intellectual footing with their (usually) younger colleagues. In any case, all recently board-certified physicians practicing in life-critical specialties must complete 40 hours per year of specialty-specific training. The Texas Medical Association can be asked to designate which specialties are life-critical, but at a minimum I would suggest cardiovascular disease (and subspecialties), internal medicine, critical-care medicine, infectious disease, and medical oncology.

You might suppose that physician education, or lack thereof, has received substantial attention from the Institute of Medicine as it addresses concerns brought to it by Congress. To the best of my knowledge, that is not the case. The IOM has 2 recent publications dealing with the state of health care in this country in which it addresses Medicare's Improvement Organization Program (IOM, 2006a) and Performance Measurement (IOM, 2006b). The former tome seems to do a thorough job of addressing issues at the process level in the Medicare Program, but it lacks any focus I could find on physician competency as a measure of quality. It does lament continuing deficiencies in care transitions, occurrence of adverse events (aka injured and dead patients), and preventive care. Further issues are too many physicians in quality improvement organizations (the implication is physician bias against change), lack of transparency (keeping of secrets), and lack of awareness among patients of their rights. The second book (IOM, 2006b) is a more readable account of the work needed to develop meaningful measures of how well our health care system is doing. Here the IOM identifies "improvability" as one of its priorities. This is defined as narrowing the gap between current practice and evidence-based practice. While this is aimed by the IOM at the process level, I think the "gap" concept clearly applies at the individual physician level. The report does state that physician accreditation organizations have adopted new standards requiring professionals to demonstrate quality-related competencies; this does not specifically mean technical competency.

In my opinion, there needs to be much greater focus on physician competence. The aggregate of evidence, both objective and personal, that I have provided in this book demonstrates the compelling need to improve the competency of physicians, especially cardiologists. If this improvement happens through the board-certification processes, it will take place over decades…decades during which hundreds of thousands of people will die as the result of uninformed medical care.

Some information I have received from the American Board of Medical Specialties (ABMS) illustrates an approach this organization is taking to lack of physician competency that I feel lacks assertiveness. When I asked what is being done to compel participation in Maintenance of Certification (MOC) by physicians who were board certified before MOC became a requirement, the answer was that "Over time, we believe requirements of health care organizations, state medical relicensure, JCAHO, etc will lead to all board-certified physicians participating in MOC." When I asked what the basis for a 10-year MOC cycle was, I was told that "Most ABMS Boards had a 10-year cycle for recertification and this was continued for MOC." I asked if there was any mechanism by which the ABMS informs employers or the public when a physician decides against MOC. The answer was that "Eventually [the] ABMS website will contain this kind of information." I asked if there were any data on physicians continuing to represent themselves as specialists after their certification had expired. The answer from the ABMS was, "Not that I'm aware of." The ABMS asked if they could review what I planned to write. When I sent them the material above, they commented to me that they are "in the process of making plans" to post information concerning a physician's MOC status. They thought the word "eventually" was not what they really meant to convey in their original response. They also noted that there are activities required within the 10-year recertification cycles, not just at then end of each cycle.

In a second round of questions to the ABMS, I was able to gain further insight. I had been told that 3 members of their board of directors were non-physicians, so I asked how large their board of directors was. The answer was that there are 31 members on their board of directors. The non-physicians are an attorney, a person with business experience, and a member of a national health care quality assurance organization. In my opinion, it is extremely unlikely that patient's rights and safety are going to be a core part of the ABMS's agenda when more than 90% of their board of directors is physicians. The ABMS did tell me that of their 21 constituent boards, 3 have a MOC cycle less than 10 years. Two have a 7 year cycle and one has a 6 year cycle. Finally, I asked about information available on efforts to deal with the grandfathered physicians who have a contract with their medical specialty boards and can [and do] legally refuse to participate in any MOC. I was told that there is not a public forum where this issue has been debated. You, as a prospective patient, should have little comfort in knowing that your board-certified specialist physician practices up-to-date, evidence-based medicine. He may be grandfathered in his specialty and not doing MOC, he may be doing MOC on a decade-long cycle, or he may have lost his certification and overlooked telling this to his patients. As I have shown you, state-mandated CME is of little value because it does not require that the education be done in the physician's specialty. No one in their right mind would fly on a commercial aircraft piloted by a person grandfathered to fly forever, or on a 10-year competency-evaluation cycle. Why do we trust physicians with our lives under these circumstances?

The most efficient way to effect change is to enact legislation that requires physicians to make their competency level more transparent to patients. This means clearly informing each patient of the physician's board certification(s) and whether he or she participates in maintenance of competency, and how often. It would not be long until patients insisted on maintenance-of-competency intervals far shorter than 10 years, and they would be hesitant to visit physicians who did not perform any maintenance of competency. Leaving the physicians alone to work out their own processes for competency through their medical boards will not work. In the end we will find that it is as if we developed the ideal aviation infrastructure, and then forgot to make sure the pilots knew how to fly the planes.

A New System for Dealing with Physician Errors

Perhaps a year or 2 after Alex died, I had become so frustrated with the bias of cardiologists who were reviewing his medical records that I sought to have the Cleveland Clinic look at his records. They promoted a service of having their expert physicians give their opinion of diagnosis and treatment based on patient records they are sent. As I was discussing this possibility with their personnel, it became clear that they would *not* look at medical records of dead people. My chance to get an unbiased opinion was defeated.

In December 2006, during my younger son's visit to a pediatric cardiologist who readily recognized, from 2 of Alex's ECGs, that my older son most likely had LQTS, the means to hold physicians accountable for their errors suddenly occurred to me. The fundamental problem with the current system of patient vs. physician is that the reviewing physician knows why he is reviewing the patient's medical record. He knows that a colleague has been accused of wrongdoing and that, if he agrees with the accusations, he will be engaged in a potentially lengthy legal process and be attacked by attorneys representing the accused physician. Dealing with such attacks could require that the reviewing physician have an incredible level of confidence in his medical knowledge, a confidence that

I think most cardiologists lack in the face of an informed challenge. The motivation to find a scapegoat and side with the accused physician is nearly overwhelming. The solution to this bias is to combine relevant CME in a specialty (or board-mandated maintenance of competency) with evaluation of medical records from cases in which physicians have been accused of wrongdoing.

Here is the way such a system would work. Part of MOC and CME in a specialty should involve physicians being periodically mailed confidential sets of medical records from a medical board. Those records would originate from 2 sources. One source would be records that are created or assembled by expert panels to directly test the competency of the physician to detect and characterize medical treatment and medical errors. The second source would be records from active alleged malpractice cases. ***The source of the medical records would be unknown to the reviewing physician***. The physician would have a week to reply to the certification board on what he thinks are the errors evident in the patient's medical care and medical records. The physician undergoing recertification will be scored on the number of pertinent errors he reports in all the records he is sent. He will look for violations of guidelines and standards that apply to the patient's care, failure to make correct diagnoses, improper prescription of drugs, failure to report adverse drug reactions, failure to respond properly to abnormal clinical findings, failure to give authentic informed consent, failures in communication with the patient, and so on. The magnitude of danger for the patient caused by each error will also be reported as a factor when reviewing the record. For example, below is the way I think an informed cardiologist would have scored my son's medical records if his MOC score depended on getting it right:

Failure or Error	Seriousness
Did not follow national guidelines for potassium replacement	catastrophic
Did not make obvious diagnosis of acquired LQTS	catastrophic
Did not know that a QTc of 490 ms is abnormal	catastrophic
Did not take time to measure QTd values in ECG	critical
Failed to request a magnesium determination in timely way	critical
Ignored evidence of heart injuries from several sources	critical
Failed to perform credible cardiac MRI	critical
Failed to give genuine informed consent for catheterization	critical/legal
Failed to communicate with patient in writing not to run	catastrophic
Incomplete and error-filled discharge summary	critical
Incomplete and error-filled hospital follow-up visit	critical
Inconsistent statements in records	
Pacemaker vs. loop monitor	falsification
Need for electroencephalogram	falsification
The cardiac MRI was negative	falsification

Note that there is nothing from the pathology report since the physicians treating Alex did not have that information at the time he was under evaluation, and the pathology report on deceased patients would not be sent to the reviewers.

Once the 10 expert opinions regarding medical records originating from a malpractice allegation have been expressed to the board certification agency, that agency would take actions against the accused physician(s) and the institution(s) where he worked at the time of the errors (Table 3). Thus if errors are not reported by at least half of the reviewing physician experts, then the original physicians have not practiced uninformed medicine. If half or more of the reviewing physicians report that they are able to identify one or more catastrophic mistakes, then the monetary fines become large very quickly. A catastrophic error is one that, when committed, substantially increases the risk of the patient dying or becoming disabled. A critical error is one that substantially increases the risk of the patient undergoing inordinate pain or suffering.

Physicians finding an error during their review	Seriousness of the error (s) found	Fine per decade of lost life in millions of dollars
Less than 5 of 10 reviews	catastrophic or critical	None
5 to 8 of 10 reviews	Catastrophic	$2.0 M
	Critical	$ 0.2 M
9 or 10 of 10 reviews	Catastrophic	$ 5.0 M
	Critical	$ 1.0 M

Table 3. Example of payments when malpractice is demonstrated

In my son's case, if we suppose that he lost 5 decades of life because he could have been expected to live until he was 70 years old and that catastrophic errors were identified by 7/10 reviewing experts, then the total fine to be apportioned among the physicians and hospitals would be 5 × $2 M = $10 M. There is no nonsense in this process: no lawyers to rake physicians over the coals or demand large fees, no silly biases as the physicians who looked at Alex's records displayed, no haggling about the money involved, and no appeals. According to this process, evidence of failure to give *genuine* informed consent before an invasive procedure will be turned over to non-medical law-enforcement authorities for further investigation and potential prosecution as a battery case. Evidence of falsification of records requires submission to a non-medical law-enforcement agency to be handled as a tampering-with-evidence case.

Prescription Errors

In the brief list of errors a physician should look for when reviewing medical records, I included 2 factors dealing with prescription drugs: failure to report adverse drug reactions and improper prescription of drugs. The magnitude of the drug safety problem is staggering and demands that physicians become more involved in protecting patients. Furberg et al. (2006) cited 2 studies in which the estimate was 100,000 fatal drug reactions in hospitalized patients each year. These authors state, "Sadly, there is no evidence that the adverse drug reaction problem in the United States is diminishing." The authors are critical of the Food and Drug Administration's approval mechanisms for new drugs, but they also assert that no more than 10% of all serious adverse drug reactions are reported. Physicians as well as patients must begin a concerted effort to report serious drug reactions to limit this annual carnage of Americans. Failure to do this would be a target for legislation and review of medical records by expert physicians.

"Off-label" prescription of drugs to outpatients is another problem that must be addressed (Radley et al., 2006). This is the practice of prescribing a drug for a purpose other than its use that has been approved by the FDA. In a study of 160 commonly prescribed drugs in the United States in the year 2001, the authors estimated that there were 150 million off-label prescriptions. The kinds of drugs most likely to be prescribed for off-label purposes were cardiac medications, anticonvulsants, and antiasthmatics. Forty-two to 46 percent of prescriptions for each of these categories of drugs were off-label. *Nearly ¾ of the off-label prescriptions written by physicians had little or no scientific support for their use. Numerically, 5.8 million prescriptions for cardiac therapies written in this single year had little or no scientific support for their use.* The authors conclude that "policy makers must begin to consider strategies for mandatory post-approval surveillance that focuses on curtailing under-evaluated off-label practices that jeopardize patient safety or represent economically wasteful prescribing practices." This should be a legislative target for change.

Recent legislation in 5 states and the District of Columbia mandated that drug companies disclose payments made to physicians (Ross et al., 2007). The investigators noted that other professions such as education and law do not allow such payments to a professional who decides how often to use a product. The purpose of the study was to determine if the legislation resulted in making knowledge of such payments accessible to the public in 2 of the states. The authors note that "substantial numbers of payments of $100 or more were made to physicians by pharmaceutical companies." In Minnesota almost 7000 payments were disclosed for the period January 1, 2002 through December 31, 2004, and these totaled almost $31 million. The authors conclude: "Making these payments publicly available will require more stringent laws with clear mechanisms for enforcement."

Disclosure of Medical Errors

Direct disclosure of medical errors to the patient by the offending physician can be another legislative mandate, but it may be fatally flawed. Currently, physician attitudes to doing this vary widely on whether they would disclose an error and how truthful they would be in their disclosures (Gallagher et al., 2006a). An interesting article on United States and Canadian physicians' disclosure of errors described several simulated scenarios in which medical errors were committed. One of the scenarios involved an outpatient given a hypertension drug with a common adverse effect of increasing potassium levels in the blood. The patient began with a normal potassium level (4.0 mmol/L) and blood was drawn a week later to monitor the value, but the physician overlooked the fact that the patient's potassium had gone to 5.6 mmol/L. The patient took the medication for another week, then experienced heart palpitations and went to the emergency room. There the patient's potassium was found to be 7.5 mmol/L and life-threatening arrhythmias were found. The patient made a full recovery after 4 days in the hospital.

I think it is interesting that the most common (56 percent) statement made by the physicians to the patient about what had happened was this: "The new medicine we started caused your potassium level to become too high, which led to a dangerous heart rhythm." The "cause" was physician error, not the medicine! This was the so-called "partial disclosure" choice. Note that the patient in the scenario made a full recovery. How would the disclosure posture of the physicians have differed if the patient *had died and they were talking to the grieving spouse and children? My point is that hoping that the vast majority of physicians will honestly and fully admit their errors to patients is a pipe dream.* Laws will be needed to systematically identify medical errors and ensure that they cease, to the extent humanly possible. Apparently, this was attempted by Senators Obama and Clinton in 2005 (Gallagher et al., 2006b), but without success. Of course, this assumes that a physician has the knowledge to know that he has committed an error.

In my opinion, legislation will be necessary to transform the present physician-centered system to one that is patient-centered. That legislation is not going to happen unless politicians know that their constituents are outraged over the current state of medical care in this country. Politicians are subject to intense lobbying from physician associations, from the big medical corporations, from medicine makers, and from the medical insurance industry. Your voice must be loud enough to be heard over the persistent panoply from special-interest lobbying.

If you or a loved one has ever suspected that suffering has occurred as a result of physician errors, then you must act immediately. There are several levels on which you can act, but the one most likely to bring much of this sort of suffering to an end is effective patient safety legislation (see Patients' Bill of Rights, Chapter 11). You must support that legislation by writing your legislators and firmly expressing to him/her the urgency of passage of such legislation. In Texas you can identify patient safety legislation and your legislator on the following site: http://www.capitol. state.tx.us/. Let your legislator know that your vote for him/her depends on support of patient safety of legislation.

Once a Patients Bill of Rights has been enacted, the state medical boards must be required to send a clearly written letter to every taxpayer explaining what their new patient rights are under the changed laws and how they can file complaints about physicians or hospitals when they receive unacceptable medical care. In addition, the legislature should require, as part of high-school courses on health, a section on patient rights. ***Once the laws are changed to create a patient-centered medical system, the focus of that system, the patient, must be aware of his rights and responsibilities.*** Why are the voices of others not heard? Am I alone? I quote the conclusion from Dr. Barbara Starfield's article published in 2005 in the *Boston Review*: ***"If the government's abdication of responsibility for the health-care system has not caused a public outcry, this can only mean that the public is not fully aware of the extent of the system's failure. It is at our peril as a nation that we allow it to continue."***

Chapter 11
A Patients' Bill of Rights

The Look of a Patient's Bill of Rights

The IOM (2001) on page 63 of their book listed 10 things that patients should expect from their health care system. I am going to prioritize these from most important to least important and expand a little on each. When your right says "told," this means you are notified in writing.

1) ***Science and Education***: You shall have care based on the best scientific evidence available. Your medical care must be based on recognized standards and guidelines. If your care deviates from guidelines, you must be told what the guidelines are and why your care should deviate from these guidelines. [Note: this means physicians will actually have to know the standards and guidelines!]. If you are prescribed drugs "off label" of their approved use, then you must be told this. You shall never have a physician represent himself as a specialist unless he is board certified in that specialty by a medical certification board. You shall be told whether your physician has completed annual state CME and participates in maintenance of certification from his medical board, and when he was last recertified.

2) ***Transparency***: Your care will be kept confidential; however, nothing will be kept a secret from you. You shall be given sufficient information as defined by the AMA (1998) to allow your informed consent well before the sanctity of your body is disrupted by medical procedures.

3) ***Anticipation***: You shall receive preventive care that reduces your risk of illness; you will not have to simply react to illness when it strikes. It is the physician's "duty to warn" the patient of lifestyle choices that pose a risk to her health and to provide direction in how to manage those risks.

4) ***Information***: You shall know what you want to know when you want to know it. You shall have full access to your medical records, which shall be *offered* to you in a timely way. These records shall exist in a form that can be read by an intelligent non-physician. You shall be able to enter your questions into your medical records. A timeline for implementation of entirely-electronic medical records shall be established for all records including those of patients in

the military, government, and private sector. These records shall be designed to be placed on a memory stick that the potential patient can carry with him.

5) ***Safety and accountability***: You shall not be harmed by errors of omission or commission in your care; however, mistakes will inevitably occur. When mistakes are suspected the patient or her survivors have the right to unbiased assessment of the treatment. When medical specialists evaluate records for errors they shall not know the reason for their evaluation. Their evaluations constitute a "jury of peers" without bias. [Note: this could be combined with maintenance of certification activity]. The system of accountability shall *not* be dominated by physicians, which means that state medical boards and their disciplinary committees shall not be dominated by physicians.

6) ***Value***: You shall never be "sold" a test or procedure that you do not need. Except in emergency situations, you shall be told *all* the ordinary costs associated with your care before those costs are incurred. You shall be told the basis for all charges posted on your medical bills. You shall be told in clear language how the health care providers are compensated in the facility where you are receiving care.

7) ***Cooperation***: Patients shall receive health care that is coordinated among all providers involved. Patients shall know who is in charge of their care, and they shall have reasonable access to that provider.

8) ***Individualization***: You shall receive treatment as the person you are rather than as a member of some illness group. Your medications shall be adjusted for your specific needs and limitations. You shall be informed of how to report adverse reactions to any therapeutic drug you are taking.

9) ***Control***: You shall be in control of your medical care to the extent you wish to be. You shall be regarded by health care providers as an integral part of the team taking care of your health needs.

10) ***Access***: You shall have multiple ways to access health care beyond office visits.

Any "Bill of Patient's Rights" must include a plan to ensure that all patients know their rights. Vigorous enforcement, including criminal penalties for battery or tampering with evidence must occur.

The goal of a patient's bill of rights is to redefine the relationship between patients and health care providers so that the patient can become a full participant in his health care and in the decisions about his treatment. Patients benefit as their health care improves and physicians benefit as they enjoy improved knowledge in their specialty, less risk of actually causing harm, and less need to be cautious when referring their patients to other specialists. A patient who takes some responsibility for her own health care may be less likely to blame the physicians for a poor outcome.

The Struggle for Patients' Rights

Rights must be guaranteed by law when some of the people cannot protect themselves from injustices perpetrated by a more powerful group. In a sense, the struggle for patients' rights is no different from the struggle for civil rights. Historically, racial, gender, and physical dominance have resulted in the need for laws that protect less-powerful groups from being victimized by those with more power. The situation is no different in the dynamics of health-care providers and the patients they treat. Unethical or uninformed physicians can wield fear and sell dangerous invasive procedures to patients who often have so much less knowledge that they can hardly ask good questions. When things go wrong patients are often unaware. I have been told by a person who has a high rank in the medical care system that patients know no more than 1% of the mistakes made in their medical care. That person also noted that little is going to change until patients "raise a ruckus."

In the beginning you need to identify key legislators and physician leaders in your state. If you think you have received bad medical care, then write to the medical board in your state, and send a copy of your complaint to the chairperson of the public health committee of your state legislature and to your own state senator and representative. And make certain the medical board knows you are bringing the complaint to the attention of your legislators. Encourage friends who have received poor medical care to do the same. If a medical institution is involved, then report your complaint to the JACHO. When the investigational results are kept secret from you, raise a "ruckus" Demand transparency in the system of accountability. Demand that the health care system give you the rights I have listed above. In an effort to focus the patient's rights movement, my website contains updated information on ways to stay informed and "raise a ruckus." It is: http://www.PatientSafetyAmerica.com/. ***Ask 10 friends or colleagues to read this book and act on it.***

This is my dream for America: One day every sick child, every stressed-out teenager, all wounded soldiers, every impoverished middle-aged immigrant, every confused old man, yes even the arrogant, beautiful, and wealthy, will have access to compassionate, informed, ethical, coordinated, affordable and timely health care.

References

Adams, D (2003) Doctors resigned to public Web profiles. Amednews.com The Newspaper for America's Physicians @ ama-assn.org/amednews/2003/05/05/prsa0505.htm (accessed 24 May 2005)

Alexander, KP, AY Chen, MT Roe, et al. (2005) Excess dosing of antiplatelet and antithrombin agents in the treatment of no ST-segment elevation acute coronary syndromes. JAMA 294:3108-16

AMA (1998) Informed Consent. http://www.ama-assn.org/ama/pub/category/4608.html (accessed 8/28/06)

Antman, EM and E Braunwald (2001) Acute Myocardial Infarction, Ch 35, ppg 1114-1121 in Heart Disease a Textbook of Cardiovascular Medicine, 6th edition, Eds. E Braunwald, DP Zipes, and P Libby. WB Saunders Co., Philadelphia

Asch, SM, EA Kerr, J Keesey, et al. (2006) Who is at greatest risk for receiving poor-quality health care? N Engl J Med 354:1147-56

Audet, A-M, K Davis, and SC Schoenbaum (2006) Adoption of patient-centered care practices by physicians. Arch Intern Med 166: 764-769

Balas, EA and SA Boren (2000) Managing clinical knowledge for health care improvement. Yearbook of Medical Informatics. National Library of Medicine, Bethesda, MD. Ppg 65-70

Balas, EA, S Weingarten, CT Garb et al. (2000) Improving patient care by prompting physicians. Arch Intern Med. 160:301-308

Bartlett, DL and JB Steele (2006) Critical Condition, How Health Care in America Became Big Business-and Bad Medicine, Broadway Books, New York

Bashore et al. (2001) ACC/SCA&I Clinical Expert Consensus Document on Catheterization Laboratory Standards, J Amer. Coll. Card. 37:2170-2214

Bedell, SE, DC Deitz, D Leeman, and TL Delbanco (1991) Incidence and characteristics of preventable iatrogenic cardiac arrests. JAMA 265:2815

Berwick, DM, DR Calkins, CJ McCannon, and AD Hackbarth (2006) The 100,000 lives campaign: Setting a goal and a deadline for improving health care quality. JAMA 295: 324-327

Boden, WE, RA O'Rourke, KK Teo, et al. (2007) Optimal medical therapy with or without PCI for stable coronary disease. N Engl J Med 356: 1503-1574

Braunwald, E and JK Perloff (2001) Physical examination of the heart and circulatioon Ch. 4 (ppg 45-81) in Heart Disease a Textbook of Cardiovascular Medicine, 6th edition, Eds. E Braunwald, DP Zipes, and P Libby. WB Saunders Co., Philadelphia

Brennan, TA, A Gawande, E Thomas, D Studdert (2005) Accidental deaths, saved lives, and improved quality. N Engl J Med 353:1405-09

Brennan, TA, RI Horwitz, FD Duffy, et al. (2004) The role of physician specialty board certification status in the quality movement. JAMA 292: 1038-1043

147

Brueck, M, W Kramer and J Ludwig (2004) Images in Cardiology: Accidental perforation of the left ventricle during angiography. *Clin. Cardiol* 27:222

Calkins H and DP Zipes (2001) Hypotension and Syncope, Ch. 27 (ppg 932-49) in *Heart Disease a Textbook of Cardiovascular Medicine*, 6th edition, Eds. E Braunwald, DP Zipes, and P Libby. WB Saunders Co., Philadelphia

Casebeer, L, RE Kristofco, S Strasser, et al. (2004) Standardizing evaluation of on-line continuing medical education: Physician knowledge, attitudes, and reflection on practice. *J Contin Educ Health Prof* 24:68-75

Castellanos, A, A Interian, Jr., RJ Myerburg (2001) The resting electrocardiogram. Ch. 11 (ppg 282-314) in Hurst's the Heart, 10th Ed., Eds: Furster, V, RW Alexander, RA O'Rourke, et al., McGraw-Hill Medical Pub. Div., New York

Chou, T-C and TK Knilaus (1996) *Electrocardiography in Clinical Practice, Adult and Pediatric*, 4th Ed. W.B. Saunders Co., Philadelphia

Choudhry, NK, RH Fletcher and SB Soumerai (2005) Systematic review: The relationship between clinical experience and quality of health care. *Ann Intern Med* 142:260-73

Choy, AM, CC Lang, DM Chomsky et al. (1997) Normalization of acquired QT prolongation in humans by intravenous potassium, *Circulation* 96:2149-54

Clayman, CC [medical editor] (1989) *Your Heart. AMA Home Library*, Reader's Digest Association, Inc., Pleasantville, NY

Cohn JN, PR Kowey, PK Whelton, and M Prisant (2000) New guidelines for potassium in clinical practice: A contemporary review by the National Council on Potassium Replacement in Clinical Practice. *Arch. Int. Med.* 160:2429-36

Davidson CJ and RO Bonow (2001) Cardiac catheterization, Ch. 11 (ppg 359-386) in *Heart Disease a Textbook of Cardiovascular Medicine*, 6th edition, Eds. E Braunwald, DP Zipes, and P Libby. WB Saunders Co., Philadelphia

Davis, D, MA O'Brien, N Freemantle et al. (1999) Impact of formal continuing medical education: do conferences, workshops, rounds, and other traditional continuing education activities change physician behavior or health outcomes? JAMA 282:867-74

Davis, DA, PE Mazmanian, M Fordis, et al. (2006) Accuracy of physician self-assessment compared with observed measures of competence, a systemic review. JAMA 296: 1094-110

Davis, DA, MA Thomson, AD Oxman and RB Hayes (1995) Changing physician performance: A systematic review of the effect of continuing medical education strategies. JAMA 274:700-5

Davis, DA and A Taylor-Vaisey (1997) Translating guidelines into practice: A systematic review of theoretic concepts, practical experience and research evidence in the adoption of clinical practice guidelines. CMAJ 157:408-16

Day, CP, JM McComb, RW Campbell (1990) QT dispersion: An indication of arrhythmia risk in patients with long QR intervals. Br Heart J 63:342-4

Eckart, RE, SL Scoville, CL Campbell, et al. (2004) Sudden death in young adults: A 25-year review of autopsies in military recruits. Ann Intern Med. 141: 829-34

Environmental Protection Agency (2001) Health Effects Testing Guidelines, Subpart C-Subchronic Exposure, 40 CFR798.2450

Farnow, GC CW Yancy, and JT Heywood (2005) Adherence to heart failure quality-of-care indicators in US hospitals. Ann Intern Med 165:1469-77

Freedman, JE, RC Becker, JE Adams, et al. (2002) Medication errors in acute cardiac care. Circulation 106:2623

Friedrich, MG, O Strohm, J Schulz-Menger et al (1998) Contrast media-enhanced magnetic resonance imaging visualizes myocardial changes in the course of viral myocarditis, Circulation 99:458-9

Furberg, CD, AA Levin, PA Gross, et al. (2006) The FDA and drug safety. Arch Intern Med 166: 1938-1942

Gallagher, TH, JM Garbutt, AD Waterman, et al. (2006a) Choosing your words carefully, how physicians would disclose harmful medical errors to patients. Arch Intern Med 166: 1585-1593

Gallagher, TH, AD Waterman, JM Garbutt, et al. (2006b) US and Canadian physician's attitudes and experiences regarding disclosing errors to patients. Arch Intern Med 166: 1605-1611

Gennari, FJ (1998) Hypokalemia. New Engl J Med 339:451-8

Gershlick, AH, A Stephens-Lloyd, S Hughes, et al. (2005) Rescue angioplasty after failed thrombolytic therapy for acute myocardial infarction. N Engl J Med 353:2758-68

Gheorghiade, M, WA Gattis, and CM O'Conner (2002) Treatment gaps in the pharmacologic management of heart failure. Rev Cardiovasc Med. 3:S11-S19

Gibbons, RJ, J Abrams, K Chatterjee, et al. (2003) ACC/AHA 2002 guideline update for the management of patients with chronic stable angina-summary article. *J Am Col Cardiol* 41: 159-168

Gravanis, MB and NH Sternby (1991) Incidence of myocarditis. A 10-year autopsy study from Malmo, Sweden. *Arch Pathol Lab Med* 115:390-2

Hark, L and D Deen (1999) Taking a nutrition history: A practical approach for family physicians. American Family Physician 59 (March 15, 1999) accessed 1/23/07 at http://wwww.aafp.org/afp/990315ap/1521.html

Harrison, EE (2001) New approaches to coronary angiography. Conference presentation, September 26, 2001, http://cardiaccarecritique.com/pages/NewApproaches.html Accessed September 20, 2005

Harvard School of Public Health (2006) Press Release: Monitoring system needed to prevent safety hazard of problem physicians.

Hochman, JS and PG Steg (2007) Does preventive PCI work? *N Engl J* Med 356: 1572-4

Higashi, T, PG Shekelle, JL Adams, et al. (2005) Quality of care is associated with survival in vulnerable older adults. *Ann Intern Med* 143:274-81

Huikuri, HV, A Castellanos, and RJ Myerburg (2001) Sudden death due to cardiac arrhythmias. *N Engl J Med* 345: 1473-1482

IOM (Institute of Medicine) (2000) *To Err is Human, Building a Safer Health Care System*, National Academy of Sciences, National Academy Press, Washington, DC

IOM (Institute of Medicine (2001) *Crossing the Quality Chasm: A New Health System for the 21st Century*, National Academy of Sciences, National Academy Press, Washington, DC

IOM (Institute of Medicine) (2006a) *Medicare's Quality Improvement Program: Maximizing Potential,* National Academy of Sciences, National Academy Press, Washington, DC

IOM (Institute of Medicine) (2006b*) Performance Measurement: Accelerating Improvement,* National Academy of Sciences, National Academy Press, Washington, DC

Isner, JM, HE Sours, AL Paris, et al. (1979) Sudden, unexpected death in avid dieters using the liquid-protein-modified-fast diet, observations in 17 patients and the role of the prolonged QT interval. *Circulation* 60: 1401-12

Johnson, DA, DL Austin and JN Thompson (2005) Role of state medical boards in continuing medical education. *J Contin Educ Health Prof* 25:183-9

Kern, MJ, M Cohen, JD Tally, et al. (1990) Early ambulation after 5 French diagnostic cardiac catheterization: Results of a multicenter trial. *J Am Col Cardiol* 15:1475-83

Khan, IA (2002) Long QT syndrome: Diagnosis and management. *Am. Heart J.* 143:7-14

Knochel, JP, LN Dotin, and RJ Hamburger (1972) Pathophysiology of intense physical conditioning in a hot climate. *J. Clin. Invest.* 51:242-55

Krahn, AD, GJ Klein, C Norris, and R Yee (1995) The etiology of syncope in patients with negative tilt table and electrophysiological testing. *Circulation* 92:1819-1824

Kruyer, WB, GW Gray, and CJ Leding (2002) Ch.14 (ppg 333-361) in *Fundamentals of Aerospace Medicine*, Eds. RL Dehart and JR Davis, Lippincott Williams and Wilkins, Philadelphia

Lazarou, J, BH Pomerantz, and PN Corey (1998) Incidence of adverse drug reactions in hospitalized patients-A meta-analysis of prospective studies. *JAMA* 279:1200-5

Leach, DC and I Philibert (2006) High-quality learning for high-quality health care. *JAMA* 296: 1132-1143

Leape, LL and DM Berwick (2005) Five years after To Err is Human, *JAMA* 293:2384-90

Leape, LL and JA Fromson (2006) Problem doctors: Is there a system-level solution? *Ann Intern Med* 144:107-15

Lee, C, W Chow, O Kwok et al. (2000) Experience with 4 French catheters for outpatient coronary angiography. *Int J Angiol.* 9:122-4

Lim, MJ (2005) Teaching Collection: Early ambulation strategies with contrast management. *J Invasive Cardiology* 17: 42-44

Longo, DR, JE Hewett, B Ge, and S Schubert (2005) The long road to patient safety: a status report on patient safety systems. *JAMA* 294: 2858-65

Marine, JE, TW Smith, and KM Monahan (2001) High-grade atrioventricular block caused by His-Purkinje injury during contrast left ventriculography. *Circulation* 104: 77-8

Ma, J, NL Sehgal, JZ Ayanian, et al. (2005) National trends in statin use by coronary heart disease risk category. *PLOS Medicine*: 2: 434-40

Maron, BJ, J. Shirani, LC Poliac, et al. (1996) Sudden death in young competitive athletes. *JAMA* 276:199-204

Matheson, GO (2006) Who says medicine means never having to say you are sorry? *The Physician and Sports Medicine* 33: 2

Mayo Clinic Health Letter, Mayo Foundation for Medical Education and Research, Rochester, NY, Prolonged QT interval, September, 2001, Heart rhythm problems, October 2002

McConnell, MV, P Ganz, AP Selwyn, et al. (1995) Identification of anomalous coronary arteries and their anatomic course by magnetic resonance coronary angiography. *Circulation* 92: 3158-62

Mergner, WJ, N Nugyen, and RG David (1984) Cardiorenal pathology in hypokalemic patients. In Whelton, PK, A Whelton, and WB Waller (Eds) *Potassium in Cardiovascular and Renal Medicine*, ppg 143-167, Marcel Dekker Inc., New York

Mirvis, DM and AL Goldberger (2001) Electrocardiography, Ch. 5 (ppg 82-128) in *Heart Disease a Textbook of Cardiovascular Medicine*, 6th edition, Eds. E Braunwald, DP Zipes, and P Libby. WB Saunders Co., Philadelphia

Mitty, HA (2003) Advances in angiography and their impact on endocascular therapy. *The Mount Sinai J Med.* 70:359-363

Myerburg, RJ, KM Kessler, AL Bassett, and A Castellanos (1989) A biological approach to sudden cardiac death: Structure, function and cause. *Am J Cardiol.* 63:1512-6

Myerburg, RJ and A Castellanos (1997) Cardiac arrest and sudden cardiac death, Chapter 24 in *Heart Disease A Textbook of Cardiovascular Medicine*, 5th edition, Ed. E. Braunwald, WB Saunders Co., Philadelphia

Myerburg, RJ and A Castellanos (2001) Cardiac Arrest and Sudden Cardiac Death, Ch 26 in *Heart Disease a Textbook of Cardiovascular Medicine*, 6th edition, Eds. E Braunwald, DP Zipes, and P Libby. WB Saunders Co., Philadelphia

Moss, AJ (1993) Measurement of the QT interval and the risk associated with QTc interval prolongation: A Review. *Am J Cardiol* 72:23B-25B

Netter, FH and FF Yonkman (1969) The CIBA Collection of Medical Illustrations, Volume 5: HEART. CIBA Pharmaceutical Company, Summit, NJ

Nuebauer, RL (2006) Paranoia over privacy. *Ann Intern Med* 145: 228-229

Olgin, JE and DP Zipes (2001) Specific Arrhythmias: diagnosis and treatment, Ch. 25 (815-889) in *Heart Disease a Textbook of Cardiovascular Medicine*, 6th edition, Eds. E Braunwald, DP Zipes, and P Libby. WB Saunders Co., Philadelphia

Perkiomaki, JS, HV Huikuri, JM Koistinen et al. (1997) Heart rate variability and dispersion of QT interval in patients with vulnerability to ventricular tachycardia and ventricular fibrillation after previous myocardial infarction, *J Am Col Cardiol* 30:1331-8

Phillips, DP, N Christenfeld and LM Glynn (1998) Increase in U.S. medication-error deaths between 1983 and 1993. *Lancet* 351:643-4

Phillips, M, M Robinowitz, JR Higgins et al. (1986) Sudden cardiac death in Air Force recruits, A 20-year review. *JAMA* 256:2696-2699

Post, JC, AC van Rossum, JGF Bronzwaer, et al. (1995) Magnetic resonance angiography of anomalous coronary arteries. *Circulation* 92: 3163-71

Puffer, JC (2002) The athletic heart syndrome. *The Physician and Sports Medicine* 7:41-7

Radley, DC, SN Finkelstein, RS Stafford (2006) Off-label prescribing among office based physicians. *Arch Intern Med* 166: 1021-1026

Ribicoff, A with P Danaceau (1972) *The American Medical Machine*, Harrow Books, Harper and Row, Publishers, New York

Richardson, DR, DC Randall and DF Speck (1998) Cardiac electrophysiology and the electrocardiogram, Ch. 9 (ppg 73-118) in *Cardiopulmonary System*, Fence Creek Publishing, Madison, CT

Ross, JS, JE Lackner, P Lurie, et al. (2007) Pharmaceutical company payments to physicians: Early experiences with disclosure laws in Vermont and Minnesota. *JAMA* 297: 1216-1233

Rowe, WJ (1992) Extraordinary unremitting endurance exercise and permanent injury to normal heart. *The Lancet* 340:712-4

Rowland, TW (1999) Screening for risk of cardiac death in young athletes. *Sports Science Exchange* 12: 1-6

Schrader, GS, CO Pickett, WD Salmon (1937) Symptomatology and pathology of potassium and magnesium deficiencies in the rat. *J Nutr* 14:15-21 (cited in Tepper et al., 1990)

Schwartz, PJ, AJ Moss, GM Vincent, and RS Crampton (1993) Diagnostic criteria for the long QT syndrome: An Update. *Circulation* 88:782-4

Schwartz, PJ, SG Priori, and C Napolitano (2000) The long QT syndrome. Ch 68 (ppg 597-615) in *Cardiac Electrophysiology: From Cell to Bedside*. 3rd ed. Eds. Zipes, DP and J Jalife, WB Saunders Co., Philadelphia, PA

Schoen, C, R Osborn, PT Huynh, et al. (2005) Taking the pulse of health care systems: Experiences of patients with health problems in six countries, *Health Affairs* W5:509-525

Seelig, MS (1980) Magnesium Deficiency in the Pathogenesis of Heart Disease, Ch 7 in *Magnesium Deficiency in the Pathogenesis of Disease* by MS Seelig. Find at: http://www.mgwater.com/calc.shtml

Sequist, TD, R Marshall, S Lampert, et al. (2006) Missed opportunities in the primary care management of early acute ischemic heart disease. *Arch Intern Med* 166: 2237-2243

Sica, DA, AD Struthers, WC Cuschman, et al. (2002) Importance of potassium in cardiovascular disease. *J Clin Hypertens* 4:198-206

Society of Toxicology (2005) Roundtable Session: Electrocardiography safety evaluation studies-New techniques and approaches, 44th Annual Meeting, New Orleans, LA, March 6-10, 2005

Spivey, BE (2005) Continuing medical education in the United States: why it needs reform and how we propose to accomplish it. Con joint committee on CME. Reforming and repositioning CME. *J Contin Educ Health Prof* 25: 134-144

Starfield, B (2000) Is US health really the best in the world? *JAMA* 284:483-5

Sugiyama, S, T Takamura, Y Hanaki, et al. (1988) Failure of beta-blocking agent to prevent epinephrine-induced myocardial injury in dogs with hypokalemia. *Res Comm Chem Pathol Pharm* 62: 407-418

Tadros, GM, JW Oren, and JM Costello (2002) Syncope in young patients II: Presentation and management of specific causes of syncope. *Hospital Physician*, May 2002, 61-67

Tamura, M, H Oda, T Miida, et al. (1993) Coronary perforation to the left ventriclar cavity by a guide wire during coronary angioplasty. *Jpn Heart* J 34: 633-7

Tepper, SH, PA Anderson, and WJ Mergner (1990) Recovery of heart tissue following focal injury induced by dietary restriction of potassium. *Path Res Pract* 186:265-282

Tsuji, H, FJ Venditti, JC Evans, MG Larson, and D Levy (1994) The associations of levels of serum potassium and magnesium with ventricular premature complexes (the Framingham heart study). *Am J Cardiol* 74:232-5

Van Camp, SP and JH Choi (1988) Exercise and sudden death. *The Physician and Sports Medicine* 16: 49-52

Vincent, GM (1998) Sudden death in a young athelete. *The Physician and Sports Medicine* 26: 59-62

Vukanovic-Criley, JM, S Criley, CM Warde et al. (2006) Competency on cardiac examination skills in medical students, trainees, physicians, and faculty. *Arch Intern Med* 166: 610-6

Weingert SN, RM Wilson, RW Gibberd, and B Harrison (2000) Epidemiology of medical error. *BMJ* 320:774-7

Wellens, HJJ and AP Gorgels (2004) The electrocardiogram 102 years after Einthoven. *Circulation* 109: 562-4

Wollschlaeger, B (2006) Save 100,000 lives lives warrant a second look. Letter posted July5, 2006 at http://floridadocs.blogspot.com

Wilkerson, JT (1995) Other cardiomyopathies, ppg 888-923 in *Cardiovascular Medicine*, Eds. JT Wilkerson and JN Cohn, Churchill Livingstone, New York

Williams, SV (2005) Editorial: Improving patient care can set your brain on fire. *Ann Intern Med* 143:305-6

Wilson, JF (2006) Patient counseling education: should doctors be doing more? *Annals Internal Medicine* 144: 621-24

Zipes, DP, JP DiMarco, PC Gillette, et al. (1995) Guidelines for clinical intracardiac electrophysiologic and catheter ablation procedures. *J Am. Coll. Cardiol.* 26:555

Printed in the United States
89320LV00003B/274/A